QUALITATIVE RESEARCH

in the Health Professions

QUALITATIVE RESEARCH

in the Health Professions

William A. Pitney, EdD, ATC, FNATA
Professor
Department of Kinesiology and Physical Education
Northern Illinois University
DeKalb, Illinois

Jenny Parker, EdD
Associate Professor
Department of Kinesiology and Physical Education
Northern Illinois University
DeKalb, Illinois

Stephanie Mazerolle Singe, PhD, ATC, FNATA
Associate Professor
Department of Kinesiology
University of Connecticut
Storrs, Connecticut

Kelly Potteiger, PhD, ATC
Professor of Athletic Training
School of Nursing & Health Sciences
North Park University
Chicago, Illinois

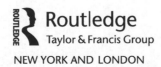

Routledge
Taylor & Francis Group

NEW YORK AND LONDON

First published 2020 by SLACK Incorporated

Published 2024 by Routledge
605 Third Avenue, New York, NY 10158

and by Routledge
4 Park Square, Milton Park, Abingdon, Oxon, OX14 4RN

Routledge is an imprint of the Taylor & Francis Group, an informa business

Library of Congress Cataloging-in-Publication Data
Names: Pitney, William A., 1965- author. | Parker, Jenny, 1964- author. |
    Mazerolle, Stephanie M., 1978- author. | Potteiger, Kelly, author.
Title: Qualitative research in the health professions / William A. Pitney,
    Jenny Parker, Stephanie M. Mazerolle Singe, Kelly Potteiger.
Description: Thorofare, NJ : SLACK Incorporated, [2020] | Includes
    bibliographical references and index.
Identifiers: LCCN 2019041519 (print) | ISBN 9781630915964 (paperback)
Subjects: MESH: Qualitative Research | Research Design | Health Services
    Research
Classification: LCC RA371 (print) | NLM W 20.5 | DDC
    362.1072/3--dc23
LC record available at https://lccn.loc.gov/2019041519

Cover Artist: Justin Dalton

ISBN: 9781630915964 (pbk)
ISBN: 9781003526100 (ebk)

DOI: 10.4324/9781003526100

DEDICATION

To Lisa, Liam, and Quin—my true north.

—W. A. Pitney

To Diane, Logan, Jane, and Jen. You keep me grounded and remind me of what is truly important—family, love, and laughter.

—J. Parker

To my two sons, husband, and family. Thank you for your endless support, encouragement, and reason to stay grounded.

—S. Mazerolle Singe

I dedicate this book to my dad, Stanley Post, who would have loved to read it. Also, to my mom, Anne, who is my biggest supporter; my husband, Adam, who is my constant; and my son, Jack, who is my heart.

—K. Potteiger

CONTENTS

ACKNOWLEDGMENTS

We would like to thank our students, who are the central focus for us as scholars. Special thanks to Mr. Brien Cummings and the staff at SLACK Incorporated for their belief in this expanded edition and for their guidance and support.

—W. A. Pitney, J. Parker, S. Mazerolle Singe, and K. Potteiger

Special thanks to Paul Ilsley for showing me the value of qualitative research. I'm thankful for my family, who always puts a smile on my face. To my co-authors, thank you for being great colleagues and always willing to listen, share, explore, and write.

—W. A. Pitney

Thanks to Judy P., Larry, Patt, and Judy M. for providing me with such a great start to my qualitative voyage.

To my co-authors, thank you for sharing your vision, time, and expertise; it has been my pleasure to be part of this team. And finally, I thank the people whose love and encouragement know no bounds: my family and friends on both sides of the Atlantic; I could not have made this journey without you.

—J. Parker

To Bill Pitney, thank you for seeing my potential and sharing your wisdom and empowering me to succeed. To my past and current students, who have the same passion for qualitative research, thank you for being a sounding board and champions for the qualitative research paradigm. To my sons, Camden and Beckett, you are my everything, and I am blessed to be your mom. To my husband, Tony, you are my true north, and I appreciate all of your support, encouragement, and unconditional love, which inspire me to reach great heights. Mom and Dad, thank you for believing in me from day one.

—S. Mazerolle Singe

Thank you to my co-author, Bill Pitney, for teaching me the ways of qualitative inquiry. And a special thanks to AJP and JAP who are my JAM.

—K. Potteiger

ABOUT THE AUTHORS

William A. Pitney, EdD, ATC, FNATA is currently a professor in the Department of Kinesiology and Physical Education and Acting Vice Provost for Faculty Affairs at Northern Illinois University. Prior to this appointment, Pitney served as the Associate Dean for Research, Resources, and Innovation in the College of Education, as well as the Director of the Athletic Training Program. Pitney has been an athletic trainer for over 30 years. He earned his bachelor's of science degree from Indiana State University, his master's of science degree from Eastern Michigan University, and his doctorate of education degree from Northern Illinois University. He has practiced as an athletic trainer in the high school and college settings, as well as the outpatient rehabilitation setting. For the last 24 years, he has worked in higher education. Dr. Pitney served 2 terms as the editor-in-chief of the *Athletic Training Education Journal* and as a section editor for the *Journal of Athletic Training*. He currently serves on the National Athletic Trainers' Association (NATA) Foundation research committee and is the Great Lakes Athletic Trainers' Association Research Assistance Committee Chair. He is a fellow of NATA and, with over 65 peer-reviewed journal articles, 5 textbooks, and more than 75 professional presentations, he is recognized as a leader and scholar in the athletic training profession.

Jenny Parker, EdD is the Associate Vice Provost for Educator Licensure and Preparation at Northern Illinois University. She is also an Associate Professor in the Department of Kinesiology and Physical Education and former Program Director of the Physical Education Teacher Education Program. Dr. Parker has published numerous peer-reviewed articles, 1 co-authored book, and 2 book chapters, and has presented at the state, regional, national, and international levels. She has reviewed for several journals in the field and has obtained internal and external research and instructional grant funding.

Dr. Parker earned her bachelor's degree in physical education at the College of St. Paul and St. Mary in England and earned her master's degree in physical education teaching analysis from the University of Oregon in 1991. She earned her EdD in physical education teacher education from the University of Massachusetts in 1996. She has received the Excellence in Undergraduate Teaching Award and the Outstanding Educator Award from Northern Illinois University and has been recognized nationally for her mentoring of undergraduate and graduate students in physical education.

Stephanie Mazerolle Singe, PhD, ATC, FNATA is an associate professor in the Department of Kinesiology at the University of Connecticut. She has published more than 100 peer-reviewed articles on subjects related to work-life balance, professional commitment and retention, and professional socialization. The platform of this work is qualitative in nature. Her work has focused on determining factors that contribute to work-life conflict for the athletic trainer working in a variety of settings, as well as strategies that can minimize the negative impact of those conflicts. Her research efforts have also included gaining an appreciation of the complex and dynamic process on how an athletic trainer gains understanding of their varied roles within the profession as a means to facilitate improved role inductance and continuance.

She is the lead author on NATA's position statement on work-life balance in athletic training. She is an associate editor for the *Journal of Athletic Training* and *International Journal of Athletic Training and Therapy*. She is the co-chair of the NATA Foundation's Faculty Mentor program and currently serves on several National Committees including the Fellows Committee, the Student Writing Contest Committee, and the Free Communications Committee.

Dr. Mazerolle Singe earned her bachelor's degree in athletic training from the University of Connecticut, in 2000; her master's degree in athletic training from the Old Dominion University in 2002; and her doctorate in kinesiology and sports management from the University of Connecticut in 2005.

Kelly Potteiger, PhD, ATC is a certified athletic trainer who is engaged in both education and clinical practice. In addition to her PhD degree from Rocky Mountain University, Dr. Potteiger holds a bachelor's of science degree from Mississippi State University and a master's of science degree from the University of North Texas. Her clinical and research focus is selected topics related to athletic training education, such as perceptions of post-professional educational programs and clinical confidence. She publishes and presents over a broad range of topics related to athletic training, environmental sustainability, and creating interactive academic learning environments to promote best practices. She currently resides in Chicago, Illinois, where she is a Professor of Athletic Training at North Park University.

Contributing Author

Christianne M. Eason, PhD, ATC is currently an Assistant Professor and serves as the graduate coordinator for the School of Health Sciences at Lasell College in Newton, Massachusetts. Dr. Eason earned her bachelor's degree in athletic training from the University of Connecticut, her master's degree in nutrition and physical activity from James Madison University, and her PhD in sport management from the University of Connecticut.

PREFACE

Qualitative research has gained respect as a method for seeking insight and understanding about our social contexts. Indeed, the depth of understanding gained through qualitative methods provides meaning to many circumstances we see in health care.

As health professionals, we function in complex environments and interact with many different people. Because the majority of our work occurs in social contexts, we are constantly prompted to consider the human condition. We are required to make significant decisions and to effectively solve clinical and educational problems. Systematic inquiry certainly guides our professional practice and informs our ability to make decisions; thus, we must be good consumers of all forms of research. My colleagues and I have written this text, which is an updated and expanded edition of our original text, titled *Qualitative Research for Physical Activity and the Health Professions*, for those who are new to learning about qualitative research so that current and future practitioners can effectively understand published qualitative studies and use the findings to guide their evidence-based practice.

As qualitative researchers, my co-authors and I have conducted many studies, taught research courses, and advised numerous students in using qualitative methods for their research projects. While there are many qualitative research texts to which we can refer our students for guidance, we have observed an interesting paradox. On one hand, although many general research texts used in health discipline research courses do a fantastic job of presenting a broad spectrum of research methods, their discussion of qualitative methods is often limited. On the other hand, numerous qualitative research texts exist in the social science and education disciplines, but many of these contain voluminous information with few examples from the health professions. For students and practitioners who are new to qualitative research, it is sometimes difficult to see how the content is applicable to the contexts of these texts. Also, although some texts present introductory content on qualitative methods for beginners, they also include advanced ideology related to qualitative research, such as critical theory and postmodernism. While this content is important in its own right, it tends to muddy the clarity of the methods for those just learning the ropes of interpretive inquiry. We believe that for many students in the health professions, qualitative research methods look very foreign compared to quantitative methods that are more traditional. Thus, the reason we have constructed this straightforward text.

This text addresses many of the aforementioned issues by explaining the principles of qualitative research in a clear, concise manner and by providing many different examples from the health professions literature. The text can be used independently for an introductory qualitative research course or as a supplement to other texts for a general research course. We systematically present the content with terms that are consistent with traditional forms of research to reveal how qualitative methods frame a researchable problem, derive a purpose statement and research questions from the problem, and guide the procedures for data collection and analysis. Additionally, we provide information on how to write and present qualitative research findings. We also refer to published studies to provide specific examples and offer exercises and activities to further learning of qualitative research. We provide expanded content to situate qualitative research in evidence-based practice, as well as how to combine qualitative and quantitative methods. Our text is organized into 3 parts.

Part One presents introductory concepts of qualitative research. In this part, readers are introduced to qualitative research and how it compares to quantitative research. Additionally, we present content on how to conceptualize a qualitative study. This essentially allows a reader to dissect a qualitative research article and see how a study is organized. Moreover, this content foreshadows content in Part Two and acts as a learning scaffold.

Part Two of the text presents information on how to conduct a qualitative research study and present findings. This part includes sections on collecting and analyzing data, ensuring trustworthiness of the data, attending to ethical issues, and reporting your results.

Part Three of the text presents more advanced content, including various forms or qualitative research. Also, we present information on how to mix quantitative and qualitative methods, and how to evaluate qualitative research and how it is used in evidence-based practice. Lastly, we conclude with a very practical chapter that provides arguments for qualitative research and identifies useful resources for continuing your qualitative research journey.

Each chapter concludes with a section called "Continue Your Educational Journey," which are activities and exercises to think more deeply about the content, check knowledge, apply information, and explore additional information pertaining to the chapter. We conclude with this pedagogy to facilitate further learning of various concepts.

My colleagues and I have set out to write a practical and friendly text for those who are first learning about qualitative research. We hope you find the text both useful and enjoyable to read.

—W. A. Pitney

PART ONE

Introductory Concepts of Qualitative Research

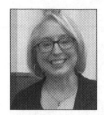

Qualitative Research in Nursing

In recent years, 2 negative health care trends have provoked concern among health care providers and the public. Beginning in the 1990s, opioid usage in the United States increased in dramatic proportions. In 2017, this worsening epidemic prompted a public health emergency declaration by the US Department of Health and Human Services.[1] The year 2017 also saw a decrease in the percentage of vaccinated children. As the rate of unvaccinated children rose, so to did the outbreak of measles and other preventable diseases.[2] This leads us to question, why are educated, affluent parents choosing to not vaccinate their children? How did the desire to understand and treat pain contribute to the opioid crisis?

Assuredly, quantitative research is essential to understanding such issues in health care. However, viewed in isolation, it is wholly inadequate. Instead, quantitative data must be viewed in relation to the holistic nature of the human experience. We cannot answer these questions through numerical data. Qualitative research provides the contextual insight commonly missing with quantitative inquiry.[3] It is this information that leads us to the question of how and why in the effort to determine how people interact with their environment as well as identify other determinants that may impact health experiences and decision making.

Many health care curriculums include traditional research courses with an emphasizes on quantitative methodology. This may leave the health care provider feeling the process of qualitative research is quite daunting. However, health care providers may find qualitative methodology is intuitive and aligns easily with the philosophy of health care delivery in which one cannot understand, diagnose, treat, or provide education without input from the patient themselves. As such, health care professionals are uniquely prepared and positioned to illuminate the human experience, leading to fundamental changes in how we engage in health care provision.

About Dr. Duncan

Dr. Heather Duncan earned a PhD in Urban Studies from the University of Wisconsin–Milwaukee. Her research involved a qualitative study of trust and social networks among women who were homeless with their children. She earned a Masters in Nursing from St. Xavier University and is a board-certified family nurse practitioner. Dr. Duncan is an Assistant professor of Nursing at North Park University and practices as an advanced practice nurse, family nurse practitioner with Lawndale Christian Health Center's mobile health team providing primary health care in homeless shelters.

Heather Duncan, PhD
Assistant Professor of Nursing
North Park University
Chicago, Illinois

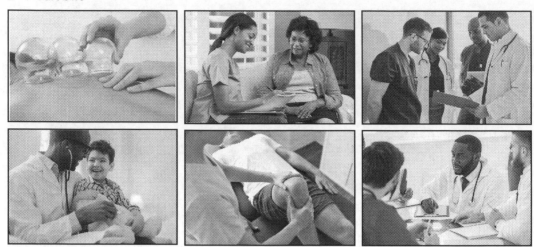

Your journey begins with an introduction to the nature and structure of qualitative research. Chapter 1 specifies both the unique qualities of qualitative research and the systematic and scientific attributes it shares with forms of research that are more traditional. Chapter 2 displays the components of conceptualizing and planning a qualitative study and foreshadows many of the aspects related to how to conduct a qualitative study

GUIDING QUESTIONS

Consider the following questions before reading Part One. They will guide your examination of each chapter.

1. What constitutes research, and why is research important in the health professions?
2. How is qualitative research defined?
3. What are the similarities and differences between qualitative and quantitative research?
4. What are the characteristics of qualitative research?
5. What are the components of a qualitative research plan?
6. How are the components of a study plan organized?
7. What is the critical link between a study's introduction and its methods?
8. What role does reviewing the literature play in the development of the introduction?
9. What does the term *theoretical framework* mean? How does it frame a study?
10. What literature would you use to guide your conceptualization of a qualitative study?

References

1. Centers for Disease Control and Prevention. *2018 Annual Surveillance Report of Drug-Related Risks and Outcomes—United States. Surveillance Special Report.* US Department of Health and Human Services. www.cdc.gov/drugoverdose/pdf/pubs/2018-cdc-drug-surveillance-report.pdf. Published August 31, 2018. Accessed June 27, 2019.
2. Hill HA, Elam-Evans LD, Yankey D, Singleton JA, Kang Y. Vaccination coverage among children aged 19–35 months—United States, 2017. *MMWR Morb Mortal Wkly Rep.* 2018;67:1123-1128.
3. Patton M. *Qualitative Research and Evaluation Methods.* 4th ed. Thousand Oaks, CA: Sage; 2015.

1

Introduction to Qualitative Research

LEARNING OBJECTIVES

Readers will be able to do the following:
1. Describe the nature of research.
2. Define qualitative inquiry.
3. Identify and describe the attributes of qualitative inquiry.
4. Compare and contrast qualitative and quantitative research.

THE NATURE OF RESEARCH

Though this text focuses explicitly on qualitative inquiry, we must first define the term *research* to provide a context for the discussion. Research is viewed in many ways. Practically, it denotes the process of gathering information to find a solution to an identified problem or answer a specific question.[1,2] We all face problems that intuitively engage us in the research process on a daily basis. For example, consider a person who is interested in improving her cardiorespiratory fitness but has a preexisting knee injury that limits her activity level. Budgetary restrictions further complicate her situation. With these problems in mind, she might gather information on equipment options and prices from fitness facilities, retailers, and manufacturers' websites. She might also ask a health care professional, such as an athletic trainer or physical therapist, about different forms of exercise. These responses to the problems make up an informal research process. A more

Pitney WA, Parker J, Mazerolle Singe S, Potteiger K.
Qualitative Research in the Health Professions (pp 3-11).
© 2020 Taylor & Francis Group.

sophisticated and scientific research process is used for complex problems and for professional inquiry.

This broader definition explains the key tenets of research for professionals. Research is a systematic way of collecting and analyzing information to answer a specific question and to add to a discipline's knowledge base. Indeed, it is a way to systematically investigate the effects of various interventions, a topic, phenomenon, issue, or problem of interest for greater understanding.[3]

The first tenet is the systematic nature of research. Researchers follow specific steps to solve problems, including collecting appropriate data, analyzing that information, and drawing reasonable conclusions from it. Scholars often question how the information gained from a study lends to their overall understanding of a topic. The second tenet is that research advances the understanding of a specific discipline or significantly relates to an area of study. Although these 2 tenets are appropriate for every form of research, the methods differ for quantitative and qualitative inquiry.

QUANTITATIVE AND QUALITATIVE INQUIRY

Quantitative inquiry, also referred to as *traditional* or *conventional research*,[4] is familiar to most students and practitioners. The term *quantitative* denotes measurement, and these types of studies represent meaning with numbers. For example, we often use patient-reported outcome measures to quantify self-reported function and well-being. Using this example, a quantitative research design may examine patients' self-reported knee function using the International Knee Documentation Committee questionnaire. With this questionnaire, ratings of function are transformed into a score of 0 to 100, with higher scores related to greater knee joint function.[5]

Quantitative Research

Many health care professionals use quantitative research to analyze numerical data, including heart rate (measured in beats per minute), blood pressure (measured in mm Hg), and blood-sodium level (measured in mmol/L). Quantitative researchers answer questions by identifying variables, measuring them, and examining how they relate to one another, or how one variable affects another. When examining the relationship between exercise intensity and blood pressure, for example, researchers may ask whether a treatment or intervention causes a specific outcome or whether a cause-and-effect relationship exists between the 2 variables. In this example, exercise lowers blood pressure (specific outcome), and long periods of exercise dilute blood-sodium levels if participants' intake of sodium and water does not match their output of sweat (cause and effect).

Qualitative Research

Although quantitative research is important and necessary, many aspects of professional and personal lives cannot be explained with numbers. As Austin and Sutton[6] point out, much of a health professional's work occurs in a "social, clinical, or interpersonal context where statistical procedures and numeric data may be insufficient to capture how patients and health care professionals feel about patients' care." Qualitative research is helpful in these instances.

Qualitative research is described as a form of social inquiry whereby a researcher seeks to understand human behavior, particularly the meaning that people give to an experience.[7] Often considered an alternative form of inquiry, qualitative research was commonly used in the 1920s and 1930s in large scientific disciplines like psychology. As the discipline of psychology expanded, the emphasis shifted to behaviorism and experimental design.[8] However, qualitative methods became commonplace in the health professions and gained acceptance in the majority of disciplines. Indeed, qualitative and quantitative methods coexist and complement one another to inform clinical practice.[9]

Researchers in the health professions have used qualitative methods for more than 30 years to expand their methodological base and to broaden their understanding of human behavior.[10] In fact, qualitative research methods are now extremely popular in the medical professions.[11] This method of study reached its current level of popularity and acceptance despite many scholarly debates about its value, legitimacy, and rigor.[12] However, many members of the health and medical communities remain skeptical about qualitative methods.[13] Devers and Frankel[14] believe one reason for this skepticism is that quantitative researchers misunderstand the process, purpose, and products of qualitative research. Thus, a look at the common attributes is warranted in this introductory chapter.

Are quantitative and qualitative research mutually exclusive?

No. Some research problems lend themselves to investigation with both methodologies.

ATTRIBUTES OF QUALITATIVE RESEARCH

Many unique attributes differentiate qualitative research from conventional, quantitative research. Numerous researchers have described it in terms of its characteristics,[15,16] assumptions,[17] and features.[18] This section identifies the unique qualities of qualitative research and compares and contrasts them with quantitative research.

Focus on People

Qualitative inquiry is extremely humanistic. Qualitative researchers are interested in how people perceive their experiences, what they believe about issues, and how their interactions with others influence these attitudes and values. These scholars study the concept of social construction, or the meaning people assign to their life situations based on their interactions with others.[19] Most qualitative researchers believe that the human perception of experience can rarely be measured and analyzed with numbers.

Use of Textual Data

Because the meaning of human experiences cannot be represented by numbers alone, qualitative researchers interpret situations with personal descriptions and accounts. They conduct interviews and use their transcripts as data. Observations or documents may also be used as data. In each case, the information is collected and analyzed by a very sensitive instrument—the researcher. The careful researcher can comprehend complex situations and identify processes, perspectives, and perceptions that technical instruments might miss.

Are textual data quantitative if they are reported in frequencies and percentages?

No. Some qualitative researchers use numbers to provide an overall picture of the data. The study's underlying attributes, research questions, and methods of data collection determine whether the research is qualitative or quantitative.

Discovery and Exploration in Natural Settings

Because the purpose of qualitative research is to better understand the human condition, another distinguishing attribute is discovery and exploration in natural environments. The laboratory environment for quantitative methods of human study, such as exercise science, is often more sterile and foreign than the environment in which people actually live and function. Qualitative researchers wish to understand the experiences of their participants in their natural settings, without manipulating or controlling the environment. For example, to fully understand the natural context, many qualitative researchers travel to schools to observe physical education classes; interview teachers, coaches, and students; and collect documents related to the study. This holistic approach deepens their understanding of human experience.

Interprets With Inductive Reasoning

Qualitative research uses an interpretive process that relies on inductive analysis. In other words, researchers construct general findings from small pieces of specific information and then thematize them, or group them together in meaningful ways, to develop the results of a study. This process contrasts with deductive reasoning, in which general principles and information lead researchers to a specific conclusion. In essence, qualitative researchers form their conclusions over time as they collect and analyze data.

Systematic Yet Flexible

The process of qualitative research is very deliberate and systematic. To ensure authenticity, researchers use specific tactics to design and plan the study, identify and select appropriate participants, and methodically collect and analyze data. However, qualitative research is also inherently flexible. It is often difficult for researchers to predict whom they will interview, which documents they will examine, or where they will conduct observations. Oldfather and West[20] compared the improvisational aspect of qualitative research to jazz music because studies often take a different direction in response to new discoveries. As a study deepens and progresses, researchers may need to collect more data or adjust the project's timeline in order to fully understand a complex situation.

Small Sample Size

Because another goal of qualitative research is to gain insight, researchers strive more for a depth of understanding than a breadth of information.[21] They rarely seek to generalize their findings, so large numbers of participants are uncommon. Samples can range in size from one person, as in a case study or biography,[22] to 60 participants with other forms of qualitative research.

Rich Descriptions

Qualitative researchers provide detailed descriptions of the setting so readers can understand the participants' experiences and the meaning they assign to their situations and environments. They also enhance their reports with quotes that showcase the participants' voices and the essence of the study's findings.

Identifies Data Patterns

Many qualitative researchers discover information about the participants' perceptions of their experiences that reveals commonalities. They group these emergent themes into categories that identify patterns of data.

Builds Theories

Conceptual model development is the process of constructing a theory, or a set of explanatory concepts, with advanced forms of data analysis.[15] Researchers theorize by interpreting data and then not only explaining what has occurred but also identifying possible reasons for the occurrence. Many researchers use visual models to illustrate their theoretical findings.

CONSIDERATIONS, CONTEMPLATIONS, AND CONSTERNATIONS

Qualitative research is not for the faint of heart. The conclusion of this first chapter presents aspects of qualitative research to consider and contemplate, as well as some qualities that may concern researchers. Silverman[18] suggests that many individuals gravitate towards qualitative inquiry to avoid statistical analysis but soon find that the process is rigorous in its own right. Researchers should be aware of the attention to detail and level of organization required to accurately execute a qualitative study. Consider also that despite the recent success of qualitative research, many scientists are still resistant to this alternative form of inquiry. You must fully understand your method and why it is appropriate for your study so you are able to defend it when necessary.

The many forms of qualitative research can confuse novices. Each variation has a unique focus, method, and set of outcomes, but regardless of the final format, all qualitative research follows the basic inductive approach presented in this text.

Finally, 2 misconceptions plague many qualitative researchers. The first is that qualitative research is often not considered a form of scientific inquiry. The second is that the 2 forms of research are often viewed as mutually exclusive. That is, a study may employ either quantitative or qualitative research but never both. This is not the case.

Is Qualitative Research Scientific or Not?

Many scholars who are more familiar with quantitative methods dismiss qualitative research as unscientific because it is subjective. Namely, qualitative findings come from interpretations of experiences rather than from measurable outcomes. These critics of

Figure 1-1. Comparison and contrast of qualitative and quantitative methods.

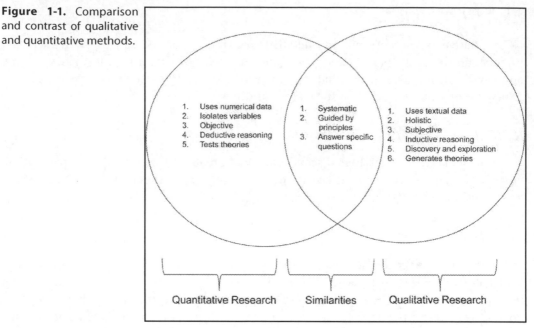

1. Uses numerical data
2. Isolates variables
3. Objective
4. Deductive reasoning
5. Tests theories

1. Systematic
2. Guided by principles
3. Answer specific questions

1. Uses textual data
2. Holistic
3. Subjective
4. Inductive reasoning
5. Discovery and exploration
6. Generates theories

Quantitative Research   Similarities   Qualitative Research

qualitative inquiry believe that the aim of research is to observe or measure a single reality.[23]

Other scholars, however, view qualitative inquiry as a form of science because its systematic approach is guided by distinct principles derived from the scientific method.[24] Shank[21] calls this process *qualitative science* and suggests that the search for meaning differentiates qualitative scientists from their quantitative counterparts.

Is One Method Better Than the Other?

These issues have led to a paradigm war among some scientists, who argue that one form of research is more rigorous, meaningful, and appropriate for the disciplines of health and physical activity; however, we argue that quantitative and qualitative approaches need not compete at all. Both are significant, necessary, and valuable forms of inquiry that achieve different purposes and answer different questions in the health professions. Figure 1-1 illustrates the similarities and differences between qualitative and quantitative research. Both forms of research can be rigorous if done correctly. Indeed, the research question should determine the type of inquiry.

If you are truly interested in a phenomenon that requires methods of qualitative investigation, then qualitative research is for you! However, if your interest is best addressed through quantitative methods, you should stick with that form of research. Keep in mind it is often inappropriate to acknowledge only a singular approach to research. All scholars have natural preferences for one form or the other, but a study's purpose and questions should drive the research method. Thus, researchers must become familiar with both paradigms.

SUMMARY

Research is the systematic process of collecting and analyzing information to answer specific questions. Qualitative research is a legitimate form of inquiry that allows scholars to gain insight and understanding about the human condition. Its key attributes include a humanistic orientation, a focus on discovery and exploration, and the use of inductive analysis. Qualitative researchers draw meaning from textual data, rather than from numbers, and work with small groups of participants. Other attributes of qualitative research include rich descriptions, the emergence of data patterns, and the development of conceptual models. Although qualitative research has gained acceptance in many disciplines, it also has many critics. Both qualitative and quantitative forms of research are important and necessary in the health professions.

CONTINUE YOUR EDUCATIONAL JOURNEY

LEARN THROUGH ACTIVITY

1. Use web-based or textual resources to explain the difference between inductive and deductive logic. How is each form of analysis used in qualitative and quantitative research?
2. In addition to the ideas provided in this chapter, give another example of quantitative and qualitative data commonly used by 2 or more health professions.
3. Use an article search data set (eg, CINAHL Complete, PubMed, ProQuest Nursing & Allied Health Source) to locate five research articles related to a topic of interest to you. Using the basic research tenets as a lens, identify which of the articles are quantitative and which are qualitative in nature.
4. Reflect on this chapter and look ahead to the future chapters, then list any questions you have about how qualitative data are collected and analyzed.

CHECK YOUR KNOWLEDGE

1. Qualitative research uses large sample sizes to generalize research findings for the broader population.
   a. True
   b. False
2. Which term denotes the meaning that people assign to their interactions with others?
   a. Humanistic development
   b. Social development
   c. Social construction
   d. Humanistic orientation

3. Quantitative research uses methods of inductive analysis and interpretive processes.
    a. True
    b. False
4. Because qualitative research is exploratory in nature, it is both flexible and systematic.
    a. True
    b. False
5. Qualitative research uses which of the following?
    a. Inductive analysis
    b. Systematic yet flexible methods, humanistic approach
    c. Discovery in natural settings
    d. All of the above
6. Which of the following is a principle related to the general research process?
    a. Methodical procedures should be used.
    b. Advanced understanding is an outcome of the research process.
    c. Only measurable data are meaningful.
    d. a and b

THINK ABOUT IT

A colleague states that because qualitative inquiry fails to identify cause-and-effect relationships between variables, it is not a valuable form of research in many health professions. What is your initial reaction to a statement like this? Explain.

Think of the personal interactions you have in your professional life, and identify a question that would best be answered with a qualitative study.

MAKE A STRETCH

Many writings exist that will help you stretch your mind and further explore the nature of qualitative research and its value in the health professions. Examining past arguments about qualitative methods that have surfaced in the health professions will serve you well, providing both an overview of the research form and a context for its current professional position.

- Clarke S. The value and contribution of qualitative research to inform nurse education and policy in response to the child's experience of hospital. *Issues Compr Pediatr Nurs.* 2014;37(3):153-167.
- McPherson KM, Kayes NM. Qualitative research: its practical contribution to physiotherapy. *Phys Ther Rev.* 2013;17(6):382-389.
- Miller WR. Qualitative research findings as evidence: utility in nursing practice. *Clin Nurse Spec.* 2001;24(4):191-193.

REFERENCES

1. Booth WC, Colomb GC, Williams JM. *The Craft of Research*. 2nd ed. Chicago, IL: University of Chicago; 2003.
2. Pathak V, Jena B, Kalra S. Qualitative research. *Perspect Clin Res*. 2013;4(3):192.
3. Stringer E. *Action Research in Education*. Upper Saddle River, NJ: Pearson Merrill Prentice Hall; 2004.
4. Erlandson DA, Harris EL, Skipper BL, Allan SD. *Doing Naturalistic Inquiry: A Guide to Methods*. Newbury Park, CA: Sage Publications; 1993.
5. Lepley AS, Pietrosimon B, Cormier ML. Quadriceps function, knee pain, and self-reported outcomes in patients with anterior cruciate ligament reconstruction. *J Athl Train*. 2018;53(4):337-346.
6. Austin Z, Sutton J. Qualitative research: getting started. *Canadian J Hospital Pharm*. 2014;67(6):436-440.
7. VanderKaay S, Moll SE, Gewurtz RE, et al. Qualitative research in rehabilitation science: opportunities, challenges, and future directions. *Disabil Rehabil*. 2016;40(6):705-713.
8. Hayes N. Introduction: qualitative research and research in psychology. In: Hayes N, ed. *Doing Qualitative Analysis in Psychology*. Hove, England: Psychology Press; 1997:1-9.
9. Clarke S. The value and contribution of qualitative research to inform nurse education and policy in response to the child's experience of hospital. *Issues Comprehensive Ped Nurs*. 2014:37(3),153-167.
10. Harris C. Broadening horizons: interpretive cultural research, hermeneutics, and scholarly inquiry in physical education. *Quest*. 1983;35(2):82-95.
11. Barbour RS. Checklists for improving rigour in qualitative research: a case of the tail wagging the dog? *British Med J*. 2001;322:1115-1117.
12. Paul JL. *Introduction to the Philosophies of Research and Criticism in Education and the Social Sciences*. Upper Saddle River, NJ: Pearson Merrill Prentice Hall; 2005.
13. Malterud K. Qualitative research: standards, challenges, and guidelines. *Lancet*. 2001;358:483-488.
14. Devers KJ, Frankel RM. Study design in qualitative research-2: sampling and data collection strategies. *Educ Health*. 2000;13(2):263-271.
15. Merriam SB. *Qualitative Research and Case Study Applications in Education*. 2nd ed. San Francisco, CA: Jossey-Bass; 1998.
16. Bogdan RC, Biklen SK. *Qualitative Research for Education: An Introduction to Theories and Methods*. 5th ed. Boston, MA: Allyn and Bacon; 2007.
17. Schram TH. *Conceptualizing and Proposing Qualitative Research*. 2nd ed. Upper Saddle River, NJ: Pearson Merrill Prentice Hall; 2006.
18. Silverman D. *Doing Qualitative Research: A Practical Handbook*. Thousand Oaks, CA: Sage; 2000.
19. Berger PL, Luckmann T. *The Social Construction of Reality: A Treatise in the Sociology of Knowledge*. Garden City, NY: Doubleday; 1966.
20. Oldfather P, West J. Qualitative research as jazz. *Educ Res*. 1994;23(8):22-26.
21. Shank GD. *Qualitative Research: A Personal Skills Approach*. 2nd ed. Upper Saddle River, NJ: Pearson Merrill Prentice Hall; 2006.
22. Creswell JW. *Qualitative Inquiry & Research Design: Choosing Among Five Approaches*. 2nd ed. Thousand Oaks, CA: Sage; 2007.
23. Munhall PL, Boyd CO. *Nursing Research: A Qualitative Perspective*. 2nd ed. New York, NY: National League for Nursing; 1993.
24. Parse RR. *Qualitative inquiry: The path of sciencing*. Sudbury, MA: Jones and Bartlett; 2001.

2

Conceptualizing a Qualitative Study

LEARNING OBJECTIVES

Readers will be able to do the following:

1. Identify the components of an introduction.
2. Construct a purpose statement.
3. Explain the significance of problem statements, purpose statements, and research questions.
4. Explain a literature review's significance and relationship to the conceptualization of a study.

FORMULATING A RESEARCH PLAN

Because qualitative research is flexible and adaptive, allowing scholars to change their data-collection tactics throughout the process, many critics believe that qualitative researchers do not plan sufficiently. However, qualitative researchers follow a planning process similar to that of any other type of study. They write proposals, follow principles, and identify strategies. In presenting this chapter, we will discuss 3 important aspects of formulating a research plan: (1) introduction, (2) literature review, and (3) methods. We present these 3 components in a linear fashion, but, in fact, you cannot formulate one component without involving the others to some extent. We will discuss this interactive process more later in the chapter, but for now we will first discuss the purpose and function of an introduction and provide tips for its creation. We will follow this by explaining the role of the literature review and offer sound advice on how best to accomplish a literature review and use it to inform your introduction. While we include some information pertaining to the methods section of a study's plan, we will do so in a manner that

Pitney WA, Parker J, Mazerolle Singe S, Potteiger K.
Qualitative Research in the Health Professions (pp 13-27).

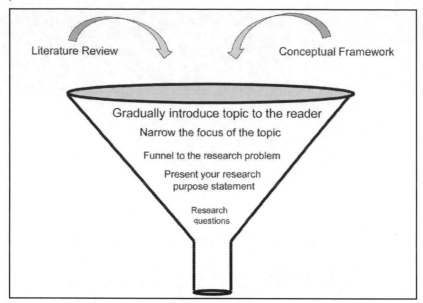

Figure 2-1. The introductory content should funnel a reader to an understanding of the research questions.

foreshadows Part Two of the text that delves deeply into qualitative research methods. Concluding information pertaining to fine-tuning a research proposal for a thesis, dissertation, or grant application is then covered in Part Three.

Designing an Introduction

A well-written introduction eases readers into your topic and helps them understand why you believe a particular study is necessary. It also places your study in a broader context. Here, you articulate your position and share critical research questions with readers so they understand what you hope to learn. Many researchers, such as Marshall and Rossman,[1] have compared a study's introduction to a funnel that opens with a wide description and then gradually narrows into a tightly focused stream of information traveling in a clear and purposeful direction. Figure 2-1 portrays this conceptualization.

Although the components of an introduction vary depending on whether you are writing for a dissertation proposal, grant, or general research study, they often have the same core components. These core components include (1) background information, (2) problem statement, (3) purpose statement, (4) research questions, and (5) specific aims.

Background Information

In your introduction, you must begin by giving your readers some general background information. The first paragraphs should orient readers to the topic and give them a frame of reference for the study. As an example, authors Lininger, Wayment, Hergatt Huffman, Craig, and Irving,[2] in their study titled "An Exploratory Study on Concussion-Reporting Behaviors From Collegiate Student Athlete's Perspectives" begin with the following introductory paragraph:

According to the Centers for Disease Control and Prevention, there are approximately 1.6 to 3.8 million sports-related concussions a year in the United States.[1] Nearly 6% of all collegiate athletic injuries are concussions,[2] with the majority of cases being seen in football.[1,3] Many studies suggest that these numbers are conservative and the actual number of sports-related concussions is much higher,[4-6] possibly as much as 50%,[1] due to underreporting of possible concussions by student athletes.

These authors provided a background and context for the study, eased readers into the material, and then ended with a statement outlining the focus of the topic—that the prevalence of sport-related concussions may be higher due to under-reporting. These authors then provided a brief overview of related studies to allow the reader to gain a better understanding of the literature associated with changing concussion-reporting behavior[2]:

> In recent years, research has sought to understand how to change concussion-reporting behavior.[7-10] Accordingly, several strategies designed to influence concussion-reporting behavior have been suggested. One strategy has been education about concussions, mainly the recognition of the signs and symptoms by the student athlete. All student athletes in the National Collegiate Athletic Association (NCAA) must participate in an educational program regarding concussions.[11] However, recent research suggests that this education may not be an effective method to improve the rates of concussion reporting.[12,13] It has been proposed to focus more on intention to report a concussion instead of concussion knowledge by the student athlete.[13] Although the intention to report a behavior does not always lead to the reported behavior, it does have more predictive value than education by itself. A second area of research has been centered around the biomechanics associated with head impacts in both football[14,15] and hockey.[16] Monitoring head impact exposures has been a recent suggestion by researchers to limit the number of head-to-head contacts that may put the athlete at risk of a concussion.[17] The NCAA[18] and many state high school athletics governing boards have additionally instituted a restricted number of full contact practices per week for football.

This second paragraph opens with a sentence that funnels the reader's attention toward previous research and the strategies used to improve the reporting behavior of athletes, including education and monitoring head impact. Finally, the authors continue to funnel the reader toward understanding the research problem.

Problem Statement

With the background information presented, we must then situate the study and provide the reader with the problem. The problem statement identifies the primary concern or issue that warrants investigation. According to Creswell,[3] a research problem "is the issue that exists in the literature, in theory, or in practice that leads to a need for the study." The length of the problem statement depends on the complexity of the issue and may range from a couple of sentences to a paragraph or more in length.

Regardless of its length, the statement must make the problem clear to readers. Researchers often articulate a problem too quickly, assuming that their understanding of a phenomenon is common knowledge. Without a broader conceptual context and scaffolding of concepts, however, it is difficult for readers to make connections and understand the problem being researched.

Using the previous study as an example, the authors presented their problem in the following manner:

> However, these strategies have not been wholly successful. Reports have shown that concussion reporting rates continue to be disappointingly low.[12,19,20] Thus, there remains a significant gap between what student athletes know about the serious consequences of concussions and what they do regarding concussion-reporting behavior.

Here the authors provide citations supporting the fact that despite implementing strategies to improve concussion reporting, the rates continue to be low. They go on to present the central tenet of the problem. The statement of the problem foreshadows the importance or significance of the study and lays the groundwork for the purpose statement and research questions

Purpose Statement

If an introduction is well written and logically leads readers to a clear problem statement, they will likely understand the study's purpose before an author makes it explicit. Even so, authors must clearly state their intentions with a purpose statement that outlines their goal.[1,3]

A purpose statement can take many forms, though it often consists of one or two sentences[1] that identify the study's central idea.[3] Take the following steps to develop a purpose statement:

- Draw the reader's attention to the statement.
- State what you plan to do in the study.
- Articulate a focus that directly relates to the problem statement and introductory material.

Drawing attention to the purpose statement is simple. Researchers often use one of the following phrases:

- "The purpose of this study is to ..."
- "The objective of this study is to ..."
- "Our study will seek to examine ..."
- "The intent of our study is to ..."

Again, using the earlier example, the authors further narrow the focus of the text to a meaningful purpose statement[2]:

> To understand this gap and design more effective interventions to increase concussion-reporting behavior, we need to better understand the perspective of student athletes who are at risk. Therefore, the purpose of this pilot study was to use a qualitative approach to reveal the beliefs and perceptions of student athletes regarding concussion reporting and the factors that may influence it.

Note that this example is written in past tense because the study has been completed. When developing a proposal or research plan, use the future tense to state your intent. For example: "Therefore, the purpose of this pilot study is to use a qualitative approach to reveal the beliefs and perceptions of student athletes regarding concussion reporting and the factors that may influence it."

The purpose statement allows readers to fully understand what aspects of the problem you will investigate and what the full scope of the study will be. Additionally, the purpose statement helps a reader anticipate the study design, which we fully discuss in Part Two of the text.

Research Questions

Once you have funneled readers through your introductory paragraphs, problem statement, and purpose statement, you should provide your research questions. These serve as the tip of the funnel, or the culmination of all the content you have presented in your introductory chapter. Do not confuse research questions with questions you might ask during an interview to collect data. Research questions are large conceptual questions you hope to answer after your study is completed.

Is it okay to phrase a research question so it only needs a "yes" or "no" response?

No! Rephrase your research questions for deeper exploration. Appropriate opening words include *what, how,* and *by what process?* Avoid *why* questions because they contain an inherent assumption of definitive truth.

Some scholars choose not to conceptualize their studies with research questions; however, we have observed that most advisors want to hear about the research questions when students approach them about a study. We believe it is helpful to provide research questions when initially designing a study. Combined with your purpose statement, they will guide your methods by influencing which participants you select, what type of data you collect, and even what you ask during interviews.

What is the difference between a research question and an interview question?

Research questions are broad and ground the entire study. Interview questions are specific and serve as stepping stones toward the answers to research questions.

Examples of specific research questions are: (1) What role do various personnel play in whether or not an athlete decides to report the symptoms of a concussion? (2) What factors are perceived to facilitate reporting a concussion? (3) From the athlete's perspective, what barriers exist that inhibit the reporting of a concussion?

In other forms of study proposals, such as a thesis or dissertation, researchers are required to include additional content, such as specific aims, study significance, and the conceptual framework.

Specific Aims

The specific aims of your proposal allow you the opportunity to briefly explain your study. Specific aims are usually no more than 3 to 5 sentences and are used to provide the reader with a general understanding of your study, including (1) what you are going to do, (2) how you are going to conduct the study, and (3) your expected findings. The specific aims portion of the proposal is important because it provides the reader with a broad overview of the project prior to describing the project in depth.

Presenting a Conceptual Framework

The conceptual framework, also called a *conceptual context*[4] or a *theoretical framework*,[5] explains the key theories or concepts that support your position. This framework situates your study in the context of existing literature and/or theory. Silverman[6] explains the critical relationship between study and theory: "[w]ithout theory, research is impossibly narrow. Without research, theory is mere armchair contemplation." Merriam[5] further emphasizes the importance of building the conceptual framework, which "draw[s] upon the concepts, terms, definitions, models, and theories of a particular literature base and disciplinary orientation."

(?) **What should I do if I do not have a conceptual framework for my study?**

Ask yourself why. If your study is unique (which is rare at the master's level and a little more likely at the doctoral level), then you may have to stretch to include other bodies of literature to support your investigation. Otherwise, re-examine your search terms and get back to the library!

Consider the conceptual framework of Podlog and Eklund's 2006 study[7] of competitive athletes' return to sport after serious injury. These authors effectively framed their study with Self-Determination Theory, suggesting that the success of athletes' return to sports after an injury depends on whether the context addresses and meets their psychological needs. This example makes clear that the introduction draws from a review of the literature, and a review of the literature helps identify the conceptual framework of a study. Use theories to frame your study even if they don't have specific names. For example, in a longitudinal study published in *Qualitative Health Research,* Thompson, Humbert, and Mirwald[8] investigated how participants' level of physical activity during childhood and adolescence influenced their perceptions of exercise as adults. The following excerpt shows how they framed their study:

> Physical activity is promoted in children because it is thought that physically active children become physically active adults (Pate et al., 1999). In other words, it is believed that physical activity tracks from childhood to adulthood. Childhood is also considered the best time to socialize children into physically active lifestyles because it is the time when the attitudes and skills develop that are regarded as important for regular adult physical activity (Telama, Yang, Laakso, & Viikari, 1997). One explanation for this belief is that the experiences acquired and skills learned in childhood physical activities facilitate similar adult physical activities as well as the possibility of adopting new forms of physical activity/sport in adult years (Telama et al., 1997). As such, early physical activity experiences have been reported as important factors for predicting adult physical activity (Engstrom, 1991).

In this example, the authors place their research in the context of 4 studies. Again, the concepts, theories, and models from the literature are used to develop the conceptual framework.

Researchers sometimes have unique ideas for studies that are based more on personal experience than existing literature. Although this practice is acceptable, Maxwell[4] points out that many scholars view frameworks grounded in experience as biased. Avoid bias by looking for literature that supports your position.

Determining the Study's Significance

We (the authors) have attended many meetings in which the first question to a researcher was, "So what? Why is this study important, or worth doing?" The question of significance emerges every time researchers raise an idea for a study. Be sure to plan for this question as you conceptualize your study.

Studies are significant for many reasons. As an example, the findings of a study may improve children's health habits. Or perhaps a study's outcome could improve a school district's funding for physical education. Maybe the research results will highlight the voice of population that is often ignored. Marshall and Rossman[1] state that studies are significant when they affect practice, policy, or theory.

A study matters to me. Is this enough to argue for its significance?

This is a good beginning, but you must stretch yourself a little bit more. Ask yourself why the study is significant to you. Once you answer that question, you may be able to place your study in a broader context.

Clarifying Your Stance

Conducting qualitative research is a very personal process. Because you will serve as the instrument for both data collection and analysis, you should share your perspectives and perceptions when presenting a proposal. In other words, you may bring a perspective to the research process that has the potential to create bias. Therefore, you should explain your feelings, attitudes, dispositions, and general thoughts about a given topic before you begin collecting and analyzing data.

Take time to search your beliefs and write out why the topic is important to you, what you think you know about it, and what experiences you have with the topic. In a sense, you need to come clean about your thoughts on a given phenomenon before you can gain true, unbiased insight from the experiences of others. An exercise like this can be helpful for every type of qualitative study. Becoming aware of your beliefs will help you keep them out of the process of data analysis. This process will also prepare you to answer the 2 questions asked in many proposal meetings: "Why are you interested in this topic?" and "What experience do you have with this topic?" Although you may not include this section of writing in your proposal document, it will help you clearly articulate your stance.

I am only interested in this topic because I need to finish my thesis. Is this reason enough?

We do not believe it is. A conscious commitment to qualitative research requires time and energy from you, your advisor, the participants, and the committee. "Just because I need to finish" does not give the research and everyone involved the respect they all deserve.

Defining Terms

As you develop your proposal, you will likely use unique terms in your introduction. Many researchers create a section of their proposal that defines special terms for readers. This section is much like the glossary of a textbook. Readers can consult it for clarification on a term or concept. It can also help you address questions about terms at your proposal meeting.

How do I select which terms to define in my proposal?

First, think about the terms that you struggled with as you developed the proposal. Next, ask an uninformed but interested party to read your introduction and tell you which parts he or she does not understand.

Assembling a Literature Review

We mentioned earlier that researchers often draft an introduction and conduct a literature review simultaneously. It is very difficult to articulate a conceptual framework and identify a researchable problem without reviewing related literature. Therefore, researchers often revise drafts of the introduction, problem statement, and purpose statement as their understanding of the supporting literature deepens. This section explains what constitutes a literature review and then clarifies which sources of literature are most appropriate for conceptualizing your study.

Reviewing Literature

A literature review synthesizes, compares, and contrasts data from published sources. It is also essential for constructing your conceptual framework. Your review of the literature demonstrates your grasp of a particular topic and your familiarity with related research. You must identify what is already known on a subject to determine whether your study is original and significant. As you begin the process, decide what type of literature to review. You should also think about how much literature you will review and how you plan to find it.

Navigating the Process

Your first decision as you conceptualize your study is what literature to review and include. Because the amount of information available in print is expanding at a tremendous rate, you can probably find published information on most topics. However, research studies must be informed by reputable and reliable sources.

When building my case, should I include a full literature review or focus on the key articles?

Initially, you should include a full literature review. You may focus on key pieces when you develop an article from your study. See Chapter 6 for more information.

Reputable and reliable sources include peer-reviewed (or refereed) articles from scholarly journals, peer-reviewed abstracts that have been published, texts written by experts or scholars in a particular discipline, and peer-reviewed papers from professional conferences. Peer-reviewed articles or abstracts are those that have been scrutinized by professionals from the field before publication. The review process screens out manuscripts that do not meet a professional community's standards of quality for publication. Many search indexes identify whether a journal article is peer reviewed, but if you are uncertain, check to see if the journal has an editorial board. If the journal lists names and credentials of editorial board members, it likely contains refereed articles.

Another important consideration when reviewing literature is whether sources are primary or secondary. In primary sources, authors present an original idea or collect and analyze the data for the study themselves. Research-based journal articles are an example. In secondary sources, authors examine primary sources and then summarize them, explain them, or compare them with other studies. If possible, go to the primary source and examine the information yourself. The danger of using secondary sources is that someone else's interpretation of primary information could be skewed, altered, or misinterpreted.

The final consideration is the age of the literature you review. Are you looking for literature published in the last 5, 10, or 15 years? The answer to this tricky question depends on the nature of your topic. If your conceptual framework is based on traditional theory such as Bandura's self-efficacy theory, you should review Bandura's original work on the topic from 1977. However, stick with literature that is more recent for contemporary issues. Go back as far as necessary to find literature that supports a compelling argument, but keep in mind that many readers want some assurance that you are aware of the latest professional developments. You should include some literature from this millennium in your review.

A literature review synthesizes, compares, and contrasts information from reliable sources. This section is your chance to show that you are familiar with existing literature related to your topic. Do not simply provide an annotated bibliography or a string of abstracts that you have written for each article or text you reviewed. This sort of review often seems like a laundry list of references with small bits of narrative about your findings intertwined. Although it is important to include your references and findings, you must work concepts together into a rich narrative.

Should I include a full literature review in my proposal or focus on key articles that build my case?

An academic proposal should include a full literature review. A grant proposal should focus on key pieces.

Organize your review of the literature with the themes you identified from critical articles and texts. This type of organization shows that you have taken ownership of your interpretations and can articulate them when questioned. Check the structure of your review by examining the opening statements of each section or paragraph. If most of those sentences start with an author's name or date, you may be guilty of constructing a "string of pearls," which lists the literature with few interpretations or thematic connections.

How do I avoid making the literature review a string of pearls?

Everyone approaches this task differently. It may be helpful to type up the key points of your articles (see Chapter 6 for a format) and then sort them into categories linked by common themes. Lead with the themes in your writing rather than the articles themselves.

Before you present the themes of your literature, show readers how you intend to organize the review so they know what to expect. The following example outlines the structure of its material. We present a brief review of literature regarding research in the area of social support networks, with the intention of specifically reviewing the coach as the main source of social support for an injured athlete, the effect of coaches' behaviors and feedback, and the role of perceptions of coaches. After addressing the coaches' behaviors and feedback, literature on the social support network is presented.

Coaches' Behaviors and Feedback as a Means of Social Support

Coaches' behaviors and feedback have a significant impact on an athlete's belief of oneself. Coaches are also considered an athlete's main means of social support (Allen & Howe, 1998; Amorose & Horn, 2000; Black & Weiss, 1992; Horn, 1984; Kenow & Williams, 1999). It has been suggested that praise and encouragement from coaches results in enhanced perceptions of physical competence, positive affect, and a desire to continue to participate in sports and improve physical skills. It has also been studied that leadership style has an influence on athlete's behaviors. These areas have been significantly studied with non-injured athletes; however, when addressing injured athletes, research is sparse. As such, investigation into the importance of and effects of coaches' behaviors and feedback on the injured athlete is warranted.

Support for the belief that coaches play an integral role in athletes' perception of ability is evidenced in many studies. One such study, conducted by Allen and Howe (1998), was designed with the purpose of examining the influence of ability and coaches' verbal and nonverbal behaviors on adolescent female athletes' perceptions of competence and affective responses to their sport participation. Allen and Howe (1998) hypothesized that adolescents with greater ability levels who perceived their coaches as giving more praise, information, and praise combined with information in response to performance and effort would report more positive affect and physical competence than adolescents with lower ability levels that received less positive responses to a performance and effort. They also believe that athletes with greater ability who perceived more encouragement, corrective information, encouragement with corrective information, and less criticism would report greater positive affect and physical competence compared with those of lower ability who perceived less encouraging information and more critical feedback in response to mistakes.[9]

Note that the anticipatory paragraph from the preceding example presents the structure of the review, and the centralized heading indicates the first theme. The author summarizes the literature without creating a string of pearls.

Some qualitative researchers believe that reviewing the literature too much can taint your analysis of the data collected later. If you read all or most of the information related to a topic before starting your own exploration, you may not make any new discoveries. This point is both interesting and important. A certain paradox does exist, because you must clearly articulate a research plan in order to navigate the proposal process for a thesis, dissertation, or research grant. You cannot accomplish this without a literature review. However, be wary of going so far with a literature review that you are unable to engage in a true process of discovery and insight that is the hallmark of qualitative research. Look for gaps in the literature that support the need for your study. Review enough sources to effectively present your proposal, but limit the amount of information you consider.

Informing Your Research Problem With the Literature Review

Your literature review is intertwined with your study and will change throughout the writing process as you reexamine your sources and revise your statements. The process is cyclical: some ideas stimulate your search of the literature, and some findings from the literature inform your study. Subsequently, your thinking evolves over time. It will take time, but the process is an enriching and important part of your research journey.

(?) *I already know how I want to collect my data and who my research participants will be. Can I skip the process of building a conceptual framework and writing research questions and go straight to the methods section?*

No! Beginning a study by collecting data is dangerous because your research will be driven by the methods and convenience of the sample rather than a theoretical base. Remember, research questions should drive research!

Methods

The methods section of your proposal should address the following aspects of your study:

- Who will participate? How will you select the participants?
- What procedures will you use to identify and recruit participants? What will you require them to do?
- Where will you collect data? What will you collect and why? How do you plan to analyze the data?
- How will you ensure the trustworthiness of your data?

Describing Participants

You must describe your participants as well as you can before meeting them. The following questions should help you write this section:

- Why are these particular participants important?
- How did you select them?
- What kind of sampling will you use? (Refer to Chapter 4 for a review of sampling procedures.)
- How many participants do you plan to use?

(?) *How do I identify the specific number of participants I need in a proposal?*

Examine your purpose statement and, perhaps in consultation with your advisor, determine the fewest number of participants needed to address your purpose statement. List this number in the proposal, but state that the final number of participants will be determined when data saturation has been reached. See Chapter 4 for a review of data saturation.

Explaining Procedures

Now that you have described the participants, you will explain in the procedures section exactly how you plan to recruit them. For example, how will you initiate your snowball sampling? You should also discuss how you will gain access to the research setting. Suppose you plan to study the experiences of students who are obese in physical education classes. How would you approach teachers or administrators and convince them to let you interview students?

? *My topic is extremely sensitive. How should I identify and approach potential participants?*

Why is this situation sensitive? Is the topic itself sensitive, or are you worried that participants may not want to disclose that they are part of the group or phenomenon that you wish to study? Discuss your situation with colleagues and brainstorm how to best recruit participants.

Collecting and Analyzing Data

The section of a proposal about collecting and analyzing data is critical. Be sure to share your intended methods. You must articulate how you plan to obtain information that will help you achieve your research purpose. Explain whether you will conduct interviews, perform observations, or examine documents, or any combination of these. You must also justify your choice of methods. Finally, if you plan to conduct interviews or observations, explain how you will record the data.

After collecting data, how will you analyze it? Chapter 4 explains that the steps of data analysis should be very clear and systematic. Inductive analysis, or the process of deriving conclusions from systematic evidence, is at the heart of qualitative research. In your proposal be sure to clearly outline the process as illustrated here by Pitney and Ehlers in their grant proposal for the study published in 2004[10]:

Data Collection and Analysis

Both researchers will conduct interviews using a semi-structured technique. The interviews will be recorded, transcribed, and then analyzed inductively. The interviewers will both be involved with the initial 5 interviews to gain a familiarity with the question posing procedures to enhance the consistency of questioning.

The inductive analysis will follow grounded theory procedures identified by Glaser and Strauss (1967) and later explicated by Strauss and Corbin (1990). Grounded theory is a systematic approach for the collection and analysis of qualitative data for the purpose of generating explanations that furthers the understanding of social and psychological phenomena (Chenitz & Swanson, 1986). The grounded theory approach consists of identifying specific concepts in the transcripts that explain and give meaning to the phenomenon of mentoring. Concepts will be labeled and then organized into like categories.

Ensuring Trustworthiness of Data

You must take steps to ensure the quality of your research. Traditional forms of research measure quality in terms of validity and reliability. Because the nature of qualitative research is different, these terms are not appropriate. We explore issues of trustworthiness in Chapter 5, so suffice it to say that you will need to comment on this for your proposal and clearly indicate what specific strategies you will employ in order to conduct a study that is credible. For example, in planning a study, Pitney and Ehlers[10] addressed trustworthiness in their proposal in the following manner:

Trustworthiness

To enhance the quality and credibility of the study, data source triangulation, a peer debriefing, and member checks will be performed (Patton, 1990, 1999). Data source triangulation (including both the protégés and mentors as participants) will be completed to compare alternative perspectives and expose any inconsistencies. The peer debriefing will be accomplished by having an experienced qualitative researcher examine the transcripts and coding sheets (which explain the emerging theme(s) as well as categories and concepts) for plausibility. Member checks will be conducted by having a minimum of three participants examine the findings to ensure that they are consistent with their experiences.

SUMMARY

In order to conceptualize and plan a study, you must write a draft of your introduction that is informed by your literature review. The introduction should include background information, a problem statement, purpose statement, research questions, specific aims, and the significance of the study. The introduction will guide your process of data collection and analysis and is informed by the themes and findings identified when you reviewed the literature. Finally, your study plan should present your methods for collecting and analyzing your data.

CONTINUE YOUR EDUCATIONAL JOURNEY

LEARN THROUGH ACTIVITY

1. Select 2 qualitative research studies and for each identify the problem statement, purpose statement, and research questions.

2. Using the following template, create a purpose statement of your own based on a problem you have recognized in your health profession:

   This study will examine <u>occupational therapists'</u> [population] <u>perceived barriers to evidence-based practice</u> [phenomenon] in <u>home health practice settings</u> [location of experience].

3. Think of a research topic you would like to explore. Write a 1- to 2-page narrative outlining your relationship to your topic. What experience do you have with this topic? Why are you truly interested in it? Be honest with yourself.

4. Select a published qualitative research article and underline the key words or terms that you must understand to fully appreciate the study. Did the authors define those terms to assist you?

CHECK YOUR KNOWLEDGE

1. A conceptual framework is based on:
   a. Existing theory
   b. The significance of the study
   c. A discipline's literature base
   d. a and b
   e. a and c

2. Research questions involve a list of questions you will ask participants in an interview.
   a. True
   b. False

3. Which of the following is the best form of evidence to use in a literature review?
   a. A peer-reviewed, research-based article from a scholarly journal
   b. A textbook
   c. A journal article that has not been reviewed by peers
   d. Objective evidence
   e. a and c

4. Which of the following items found in scholarly literature is a primary source of information?
   a. An article reviewing the research literature
   b. An encyclopedia
   c. A research-based article
   d. A textbook

5. Which of the following items is not a component of an introduction?
   a. Significance of the study
   b. Methods
   c. Problem statement
   d. Purpose statement
   e. Research questions

6. When writing a literature review, you should summarize the results of various studies in sequential order, usually chronologically.
   a. True
   b. False

7. The introduction of a study should contain:
   a. Background information
   b. Statement of the problem
   c. A purpose statement
   d. Research questions
   e. All of the above

THINK ABOUT IT

1. You are interested in studying how chronic pain patients cope with continued pain while trying to be active. What key terms would you use to search for pertinent literature?
2. Identify 2 or 3 reasons why a researcher would study burnout among nurses in intensive care settings.
3. Research questions guide a study and help narrow a researcher's focus. A researcher may use one broad research question or several specific research questions. List the advantages and disadvantages for each approach.

MAKE A STRETCH

Examine the 2 articles here to learn more about conceptualizing your study and the use of conceptual frameworks.

1. Examine the following open-access article by Ronald Chenail. The first of his 10 steps relates to conceptualizing a qualitative study and will walk you through steps to better focus your interests.
   - Chenail RJ. Ten steps for conceptualizing and conducting qualitative research studies in a pragmatically curious manner. *Qual Rep.* 2011;16(6):1713-1730.
2. Helen Green provides an excellent overview of the use of frameworks in qualitative research and clarifies the difference between conceptual and theoretical frames.
   - Green H. Use of theoretical and conceptual frameworks in qualitative research. *Nurse Res.* 2014;21(6):34-38.

REFERENCES

1. Marshall C, Rossman GB. *Designing Qualitative Research.* 3rd ed. Thousand Oaks, CA: Sage; 1999.
2. Lininger MR, Wayment HA, Hergatt Huffman A, Craig DI, Irving LH. An exploratory study on concussion-reporting behaviors from collegiate student athletes' perspectives. *Athl Train Sports Health Care.* 2017;9(2):71-80.
3. Creswell JW. *Research Design: Qualitative, Quantitative, and Mixed Methods Approaches.* 2nd ed. Thousand Oaks, CA: Sage; 2003.
4. Maxwell JA. *Qualitative Research Design: An Interactive Approach.* Thousand Oaks, CA: Sage; 1996.
5. Merriam SB. *Qualitative Research and Case Study Applications in Education.* 2nd ed. San Francisco, CA: Jossey-Bass; 1998.
6. Silverman D. *Doing Qualitative Research: A Practical Handbook.* Thousand Oaks, CA: Sage; 2000.
7. Podlog L, Eklund RC. A longitudinal investigation of competitive athletes' return to sport following serious injury. *J Applied Sport Psych.* 2006;18:44-68.
8. Thompson A, Humbert M, Mirwald R. A longitudinal study of the impact of childhood and adolescent physical activity experiences on adult physical activity perceptions and behaviors. *Qual Health Res.* 2003;13(3);358-377.
9. Borseth KM. *An investigation of the Social Support Network of Injured Athletes.* Unpublished master's thesis, Northern Illinois University, De Kalb, Illinois; 2004.
10. Pitney WA, Ehlers GG. A grounded theory study of the mentoring process involved with undergraduate athletic training students. *J Athl Train.* 2004;39(4):344-351.

PART TWO

Fundamental Principles of Conducting Qualitative Research

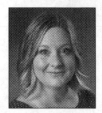

Qualitative Research in Physical Therapy

I learned the value of qualitative research while I was a PhD student at the University of South Carolina. I was lucky enough to work under the direction of Dr. Stacy Fritz who was studying the impact of intensive therapy on various neurological populations, such as stroke and incomplete spinal cord injury. Participants involved in the research completed 30 hours of intensive therapy over 10 days. Session were 3 hours a day with a goal of only 10 minutes of rest per hour. Our hope was to see improvements in walking, balance, and general mobility and we chose the typical standardized outcome measures used in the physical therapy field to do so. At the conclusion of the study, we analyzed the data to find mainly small effect sizes. We went on and published the study, which virtually told the therapy community that perhaps this intensive therapy was not worth the time and effort.

I knew our data was not telling the whole story. Daily exposure to participants and conversations with participants, family members, and caregivers painted a very different picture. We learned of many positive changes in their lives as result of the therapy, including the ability to get in and out of a bathtub without assistance, going to the rest room independently, the ability to get a drink out of the refrigerator by themselves, choosing not to use a wheelchair at a restaurant or a motorized cart at the market, even reports of improved happiness and a return to pre-injury personality. In fact, one caregiver reported the therapy as "life changing." These examples represent only a handful of meaningful changes we failed to capture and report using traditional quantitative methodology.

The incorporation of qualitative research is needed to paint a more clear and complete picture of rehabilitation efforts. Numerical data, although necessary, does not capture the meaningful experiences of those who participate. After all, if we are studying an intervention *for the people*, shouldn't we include the voices *of the people*?

About Dr. Merlo

Dr. Merlo received her BS in Physical Education from University of Puget Sound, an MS in Exercise Science and Health Promotion from Cal Poly San Luis Obispo, and both her DPT and PhD in Exercise Science from the University of South Carolina. Dr. Merlo is full time faculty at Eastern Washington University in Spokane, Washington. She also serves as adjunct faculty for Rocky Mountain University of Health Professions, where she teaches qualitative research to doctoral students. Her interests include intervention strategies for chronic neurologic conditions, as well as educational and testing practices in physical therapy education.

Angela Merlo, PT, DPT, PhD
Assistant Professor
Eastern Washington University
Spokane, Washington

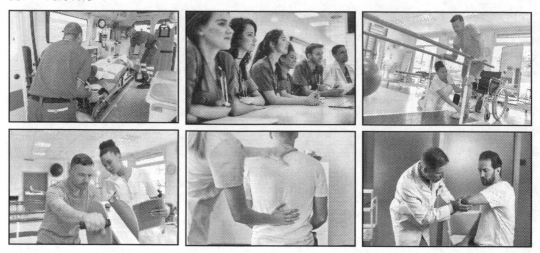

The next section of our text focuses on specific methodological strategies, including various forms of data collection, sampling, and data analysis. We begin Part Two with Chapter 3, which focuses on the collection and analysis of qualitative data. Chapter 4 explains the importance of ensuring trustworthiness in a qualitative research study, and Chapter 5 addresses ethical issues connected to the research process. We conclude this section of the text with Chapter 6, which presents information on how to write a research report; this chapter outlines ways to present results using participants' quotes to support the findings. It also provides advice about how to write the discussion and conclusion sections of a manuscript.

GUIDING QUESTIONS

Consider the following questions before reading Part Two. They will guide your examination of each chapter.

1. What are common methods of collecting and analyzing data?
2. What forms of qualitative data exist?
3. What are the 8 steps for analyzing qualitative data?
4. What does trustworthiness mean in the context of qualitative research?
5. What does the term *informed consent* mean? What role does it play in qualitative research?
6. What steps are required for the protection of a study's participants?
7. What options do you have when seeking a balance between the voices of participants and researchers in your results section?
8. How can you use participants' quotes to support a study's thematic findings?

3

Collecting and Analyzing Qualitative Data

LEARNING OBJECTIVES

Readers will be able to do the following:
1. Identify various forms of qualitative data.
2. Collect qualitative data through interviews, observations, and document reviews.
3. Outline different sampling strategies.
4. Explain the steps of qualitative data analysis.

THE INTERPRETIVE PROCESS

This chapter explains different methods of data collection and outlines the steps of data analysis. The ultimate goal of a qualitative study is to interpret your findings.

Interpretation, or the process of explaining meaning, is the underlying premise to all qualitative research, which seeks understanding about particular problems. Stringer[1] explains that the process of interpretation allows researchers to understand the experiences of participants—specifically what they feel and believe about various phenomena. Researchers gain insight from the experiences of their participants by systematically collecting and analyzing appropriate data. The outcome of any inquiry is as good as the data you collect. The first step in obtaining quality information is to select an appropriate sample of participants.

Pitney WA, Parker J, Mazerolle Singe S, Potteiger K.
Qualitative Research in the Health Professions (pp 31-48).
© 2020 Taylor & Francis Group.

SAMPLING STRATEGIES IN QUALITATIVE METHODS

Once the study's purpose, research questions, and significance have been established, it is time to select participants. Qualitative strategies rely on purposeful strategies.[2,3] Sampling in qualitative methods should be viewed as purposeful selection[3] or purposive sampling.[4] Qualitative research relies on strategies of purposeful sampling as a means to ensure the researchers can collect data to answer the study's purpose and research questions.[2,3]

Tuckett[5] encourages researchers to carefully consider participant sampling strategies with each study, as they are unique and have different intended outcomes. When choosing a sampling strategy, it is important to reflect on the study's purpose and research questions. It is important when choosing participants that those individuals who can offer information-rich data are selected. This will involve identifying those individuals who are knowledgeable about or have experienced the phenomenon of interest.[3]

Types of Sampling

Several specific strategies exist within the general category of purposeful sampling.[3] Several of the most commonly utilized sampling methods include criterion, maximum variation, typical, snowball, convenience, homogeneous, and total population.

Criterion Sampling

Criterion sampling is the most commonly implemented type of sampling in qualitative research.[6] The researcher predetermines a set of criteria for selecting participants, and this is done to reflect a particular set of attributes or characteristics or past experiences being studied. Creswell[3] suggests criterion sampling offers quality assurance in the research design of the study.

Maximum Variation Sampling

Maximum variation sampling refers to exploring different perspectives of one situation or phenomenon by recruiting a variety of backgrounds or positions for a study. The idea is to allow researchers to fully explore many facets of a problem and view it holistically. It can also be referred to as *heterogeneous sampling*. For example, if you are studying the use of strategic questioning in the clinical education setting as a means to foster critical thinking development, you may select students, clinical educator coordinators, and preceptors to better understand its use and effectiveness.

Typical Sampling

In typical sampling, a researcher chooses a participant who fits with the norm for a given population. As Creswell[3] notes, it can be difficult for researchers to identify what is typical for a certain group. According to Merriam[7] the typical sample should be "selected because it reflects the average person, situation, or instance of the phenomenon of interest." The goal is to select the average participant.

Snowball Sampling

Snowball sampling, also referenced as *chain* or *network sampling*, utilizes informants or enrolled participants to gain access to other cases or participants who have information-rich data based upon the criterion.[3,8] For example, you may be studying women athletic trainers who have left the profession. To gain access to these women, you may ask already enrolled participants for other women athletic trainers who have left the profession as well.

Convenience Sampling

Convenience sampling is a sampling process of selecting and recruiting participants based upon accessibility, ease, and speed. It can also be referred to as *availability sampling*. This sampling strategy is often used in combination with other strategies, such as criterion or snowball sampling. For example, if a researcher wants to study the experiences of women athletic trainers in the Division I setting who have left the profession, the researcher may contact a participant with whom he or she has a relationship, as she meets the criteria. The access to the first participant was convenient, but she met the study's criterion. From there, the researcher could ask this individual for other contacts she knows and shift to a snowball sampling strategy.

Homogeneous Sampling

Homogeneous sampling is used when the goal is to understand, describe, or explore a particular group's experiences in depth. The sample is often small and bound by a common set of attributes, characteristics, or experiences. For example, the number of females in athletic training who assume the role of the head athletic trainer in the Division I setting is small.

Total Population Sampling

Total population sampling includes everyone associated with a small group as participants in a study. For example, if you were conducting a case study of a unique doctoral degree being offered to a small group of students in the field of health education, you might cover the total population by interviewing the teacher, students, and department chair.

Sample Size

The size of the sample is an important consideration for qualitative research methods. Typically speaking, sample sizes are small, and decisions regarding the total number of participants included is often guided by the strategy called *data saturation* or *data redundancy*. Data saturation is the point in the data collection process where no new information is being encountered or the enrolled participants are continually sharing the same information with the researchers. Bowen[9] describes the saturation as "bringing new participants continually into the study until the data set is complete, as indicated by data replication or redundancy." Once hearing the same information over and over from different participants, it may be indicative of saturation. Determining saturation can be done as the data collection process is happening (ie, ongoing, constant comparison of the data) or after a series of participants have completed the study's protocol and the researchers evaluate the data. The latter may require recruitment of additional participants to complete the study's protocol if saturation of data is not met.

Saturation is key to an excellent qualitative research study; however, as Morse[10] illustrates, there are "no published guidelines or tests of adequacy for estimating the sample size required to reach saturation." Patton,[8] however, notes the benefits of ambiguity

TABLE 3-1
TYPICAL SAMPLE SIZE WITH VARIOUS FORMS OF QUALITATIVE RESEARCH

APPROACH	MINIMAL SAMPLE SIZE
Narrative	1 participant
Phenomenology	3 to 12 participants
Grounded theory	10 to 30 participants
Case study	3 to 5 participants (with observations and/or artifacts)
Ethnography	1 participant (with associated artifacts)

regarding sample size and urges researchers to carefully navigate sample size by the study's purpose, what will be useful in answering the research questions, and what can be done with the available time and resources.

In addition to the general principle of data saturation, it may be useful to examine currently published data within the field, as they can provide a better understanding of the common practice for sample size. Example sizes can vary. A few studies are included here with their associated sample sizes:

- Jackson[11] examined the process of resilience among post-qualification nursing students. The author interviewed a total of 10 students in this grounded theory study.
- Mazerolle and Eason[12] investigated work-life balance from an individual and socio-cultural perspective using 27 female athletic trainers.
- Reitz, Horst, Davenport, Klemmetsen, and Clark[13] examined factors that influenced the scope of care among physicians practicing in rural settings. They interviewed 21 physicians.
- Mazerolle and Eason[14] explored the work-life balance experiences of 6 athletic trainers over a year.
- Petursdottir, Arnadottir, and Halldorsdottir[15] sought to understand the perceived barriers to exercise among patients with osteoarthritis. These researchers conducted a total of 16 interviews with 12 participants, all of whom were 50 years of age or older and diagnosed with osteoarthritis.
- Thrasher, Walker, Hankemeier, and Mulvihill[16] studied the experiences of 19 graduate assistant athletic trainers as they transitioned into clinical practice for the first time.
- Flinkman, Isopahkala-Bouret, and Salantera[17] studied nurses intent on leaving the profession early in their career. These authors interviewed 3 nurses over several years.

One final consideration with sample size can be the type of qualitative design used by the researchers. Creswell[3] has shared that various approaches within qualitative research may require various sample sizes. Based on Creswell's thoughts on sample size, and having examined recent published examples (such as those listed earlier), we present typical sample sizes in Table 3-1.

Sample Accessibility

Another important consideration in qualitative research is how you will gain access to individuals or programs to collect your data. When selecting a research site and participants, you are often at the mercy of factors beyond your control. This may affect your sampling strategy and sample size. A gatekeeper is one strategy used to help gain access to a research site or participants. The gatekeeper is a person who stands between the researchers and the potential participants.[3]

COLLECTING QUALITATIVE DATA

Qualitative researchers use many forms of data. Those who are interested in learning about specific cultures might consider artifacts and ritualistic items. However, most of us use interviews, observations, and various forms of documents as data.

Interviews

According to Kvale[18] an interview is "a conversation, whose purpose is to gather descriptions of the [life-world] of the interviewee" with respect to their perceptions of events or their interpretation of the meaning of a phenomenon. In a parallel perspective, Schostak[19] adds that "an interview is an extendable conversation between partners that aims at having an 'in-depth conversation' about a certain topic or subject, and through which a phenomenon could be interpreted in terms of the meanings interviewees bring to it."

Types of Interviews

Interviews can be conducted either face to face or over the phone. Face-to-face interviews are often viewed as the gold standard in qualitative research; however, the use of phone interviews is growing in popularity as well as convenience. Also, interviews can be done one on one or in a group, often termed a *focus group*.

Face-to-Face Interviews

Face-to-face or in-person interviews are conducive to the development of a personal connection between the participant and researcher, as they can feed off the social and nonverbal cues offered. The ability to ask longer questions and engage more with the participant are likely advantages to the in-person interview. In-person interviews require extensive scheduling for both parties, require travel time, and usually cost the most.[20]

Phone Interviews

Conducting phone interviews has advantages, including logistical conveniences to gaining a geographically diverse group of participants, reduced costs (ie, no travel), and greater flexibility with scheduling.[3,21,22] Possibly the greatest benefit for a phone interview is the increased sense of anonymity by the participant, which may increase their desire to share and reflect when compared to a face-to-face interview.[23] It is also suggested that researcher or interviewer bias is reduced with the phone interview, as the participant may feel more comfortable and be forthright and truthful with information.[20] The disadvantages to the phone interview include challenges with establishing rapport, the inability to capture or respond to visual cues, and the potential loss of contextual data.[24,25]

Focus Group Interviews

Focus groups are also a method of interviewing. The method allows for the collection of data from a variety of divergent thoughts over a short period. Krueger[26] suggests that a focus group is a carefully planned activity to gather the perceptions on a specific area of study in a nonjudgmental, nonthreatening setting. Group members influence and share their experiences within the group setting by responding to a series of planned questions. It is recommended that focus groups contain between 3 and 6 and no more than 10 participants per interview session. A facilitator who is engaging and asking the questions is recommended, along with an observer, who will not engage in the discussion but will record relevant information and observations. Advantages of this type of interview are the interactions and energy gained among the group's participants.[3,26] Managing groups can be challenging, however, and can allow more dominant personalities to overwhelm the discussions.[3,26]

Interview Structure

Interview guides, or protocols, list the questions and statements a researcher will follow during the interview session. There are 3 main types of interview structures: (1) unstructured, (2) semi-structured, and (3) structured.[27]

Unstructured Interviews

Unstructured interviews take place with few, if any, interview questions, as the goal is to create a natural conversation between the researcher and the participant. Rapport often is established with ease, and this type of interview format may help with sensitive topics or those that have been understudied. The researcher must be knowledgeable about the topic and have confidence during the interview as a way to probe and ask questions to gain all the information necessary to answer the research questions.

Semi-Structured Interviews

Semi-structured interviews use an interview protocol that guides the interview session using predetermined questions yet has flexibility to allow the researcher to go off script and ask follow-up questions. This can be helpful in capturing participants' thoughts, feelings, and opinions.

Structured Interviews

Structured interviews strictly adhere to an interview guide created prior to data collection. This is a rigid form of data collection, and the researcher does not deviate from the script. There are limited opportunities to create follow-up questions or expand upon answers provided in the interview session. Structured interviews are most common in an online platform, where the questions are open-ended and the participant is asked to write their answers rather than verbally communicate them. This method of interviewing can be beneficial when there is a comprehensive list of questions to be answered.

Conducting Effective Interviews

Interviews play a central role in data collection, and thus conducting effective interviews is important. The ability to speak directly to your participants about their beliefs, attitudes, and perceptions is the best way to gain information-rich data. Interview sessions must make your participants feel comfortable and open to sharing their views; this is often referred to as *establishing rapport*. Rapport can be built upon the researcher being confident, easy to speak to and with, and neutral regarding the topic being studied.[28] Building a relationship will help create an interview environment that is encouraging of sharing and reflecting on their experiences.

The success of an interview can also be attributed to the interviewer. The interviewer should be knowledgeable about not just the topic being investigated but also the interview protocol to be used during the data collection process.[3,29] During the interview, the researcher should be clear and articulate when asking questions, but also an active listener ready to probe and follow up. In fact, the interviewer needs to be balanced, as he or she should talk only when necessary, and encourage yet make the participate feel at ease to share his or her story.[29] The researcher should show sensitivity, as well as an open mind as he or she listens to the participant share and respond to the questions asked.

Many authors have offered their thoughts about how interviews should be conducted. After careful consideration, we formulated the following discussion based upon the work of Kvale and Brinkman[29] and Creswell.[3]

Organizing Your Interview

It is important to remember that the data collection process is critical, as you will collect information that will help you answer your research question. Moreover, you have been invited to share a small portion of your participants' world, and they have offered you their valuable time. You must plan ahead to make every moment with them count and ensure that the event is mutually enriching. When planning for your interview, consider these 5 important components:

1. *Setting the stage:* Provide the interviewee/participant with a framework for the study.
2. *Building the relationship:* Set the tone for your relationship, and help your interviewee feel comfortable.
3. *Addressing the research focus:* Ask your interview questions as detailed by 1 of the 3 types of interview protocols.
4. *Debriefing:* Conclude the interview by identifying the important things you learned. Obtain permission to follow up at another time, if necessary.
5. *Thanking your participants:* Genuinely thank you participants for the opportunity to learn about their experiences.

SETTING THE STAGE. Before the interview begins, it is important to orient your participants to the interview process and share why you are interested in speaking with them. Take time to briefly explain the purpose of your study in terms that they will understand and remind them their participation is voluntary. This is often done as part of the consenting process in compliance with institutional review board procedures. Ask permission to record them and the conversation that will follow the interview protocol and let them know that they can decline to answer a question at any time. Reassure your participants that you will maintain confidentiality before you begin the interview process. Consent can be gained either verbally or in a written format.

BUILDING THE RELATIONSHIP. It is important to start the interview by making participants feel comfortable and at ease. This can be done simply by easing them into the interview protocol. Kvale[18] suggests using a series of dynamic questions to establish a positive relationship with the participant. Examples of the types of questions to ask include "Tell me a little bit about yourself," "What is your academic background?" or "Can you tell me a little bit about your day and daily routines?"

ADDRESSING THE RESEARCH FOCUS. The research is the heart of the process and your reason for interviewing the participant in the first place. Your goal is to learn information that will help you address your research questions. You must ask good questions; probe appropriately to obtain depth; and direct your participants to share their thoughts, beliefs, and experiences.

It is important to stop and think about your research agenda, particularly the purpose and research questions, before you develop the interview protocol. The literature and your knowledge as a researcher should also play a role in the development of the protocol. Interview questions are often focused on gaining as much information on the participant's experiences, behaviors, opinions/values, and knowledge as they pertain to a particular phenomenon.[8,29]

We ran out of time for the interview before I was able to ask all of my questions. What should I do?

The duration of interviews varies because some participants talk a lot and others provide brief answers. If you run out of time, ask to schedule another interview.

Questions, regardless of the type of interview protocol selected, should be direct and focused. Ask the participant a simple question that can elicit a detailed response yet avoid a one-word answer.[29] Don't be afraid to ask probing questions as a means to gain more information. It is important to ask questions that gain the "how" and use follow-up questions later to gain the "why."[8] The flow of the interview protocol is also important. Include broader, general questions initially; this can develop rapport and ease the participant into the more specific or hard-hitting questions that may require more thought and reflection. The inclusion of both open- and closed-ended questions is encouraged because each offers different information. For example, closed-ended questions are often included early to gain more demographic type information (ie, age, years of experience). If a closed-ended question is used and is not related to background or demographic data, follow-up questions may be asked immediately to ensure full understanding is reached.

It is important to pilot the interview protocol to determine flow as well as interpretability of the interview protocol. Creswell[3] suggests piloting the instrument is a time to determine its usefulness and feasibility (ie, length of the interview). Using participants who have knowledge of the topic and fit the inclusion criteria can be beneficial in determining the viability of the questions, as well as the flow and length the interview protocol may require.

The interview is off-course. How do I redirect my participant without cutting her off and feeling as though her voice is not being heard?

Although you should be wary of interrupting or ignoring your participant's train of thought, it may help to use a phrase like, "Can you relate that thought to the initial question for me?" You could also say something like, "I would really like to hear more about this topic. Would you mind if we revisit it at the end of the interview?"

In summation, interview questions can be both open- and closed-ended, but follow-up may be necessary. Present one question at a time and not multipart questions so as to ensure the participant can fully articulate their experiences. Sequencing of questions should begin broadly and then funnel into more specific, focused questions related to the phenomenon.

My participant asked me to keep part of the interview off the record before revealing information that is critical to my study. Can I use the information?

The short answer is no; however, you may ask participants why they wish to exclude certain comments from the interview and offer them reassurances about your confidentiality practices. If your participants remain firm in their convictions, you must honor their requests.

DEBRIEFING AND THANK YOU. This is part of the closure of the interview protocol. You can thank your participants for their time and communicate what happens next. It is also the chance to share the key points you've heard and learned and to clarify anything as necessary. You may also inquire whether they are willing to complete any follow-up interviews needed after the interview has been transcribed and analyzed. At this time, you can ask them to provide pseudonyms to be identified as in any research report or publication.

Observations

Participant observation is a trademark of ethnography and anthropological studies.[30] It can be characterized as a systematic and detailed look at interactions, behaviors, and events within an environmental setting under investigation. Observations allow the researcher to be active in the research process, allowing them to learn about the activities and experiences of the people under study in their natural environment.[30] Answering a descriptive research question, building a theory, or generating or testing hypotheses is best done with participant observations.[30]

Unlike an interview, during an observation the researcher takes field notes as a means to capture what he or she is seeing and witnessing. A challenge in participant observation is missing something of value while note taking. To reduce this, researchers sometimes video-record the environment and the participant in addition to taking field notes. Observations are an immersive process and can be time intensive. Thus, to be effective, the researcher must decide how to record the observations, determine what needs to be observed (ie, body language, frequency of interactions), and what role is important to take during the observations (ie, silent observer or active participant).

Much like the other methods of collecting data, there is speculation that a researcher in participant observations cannot be both objective and subjective. However, researcher bias can be curbed if the researcher is able to reflect on one's biases and own personal experiences and beliefs prior to observation.[31] Additionally, reducing bias during the data collection process can be done when the researcher provides quality documentation, which can be accomplished by keeping detailed field notes. Other documentation can include videotapes and artifacts.

Participant observation is more difficult than a simple observation, as it is important to observe as well as record the activities that are occurring during the period of data collection. Like other methods of data collection, the researcher must establish rapport and a relationship that can offer sharing of information; however, the presence of the researcher must not influence the normal activities or interactions of the participant while being studied.

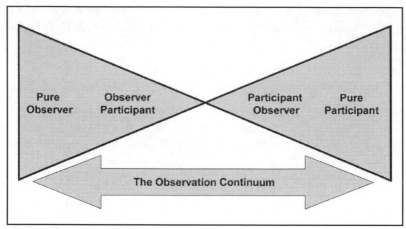

Figure 3-1. The observation continuum.

How to Observe

General guidelines for conducting an observation include the following[30,32]:

- Be inconspicuous in dress and actions.
- Become familiar with the setting before collecting data.
- Be discreet but open regarding the reason for the observation.
- Be cognizant, pay attention, and try to see the whole picture while avoiding tunnel vision.
- Focus on the interactions while actively observing and listening intently.

You will need to choose how to perform your observations. Merriam[7] states that observations can be viewed on a continuum that ranges from participatory to nonparticipatory (Figure 3-1). Similarly, Mills[33] explains the role of the observer as ranging from active observation to passive observation. Each form has advantages and disadvantages.

If you choose to observe passively, you will have time to document events as they occur. A disadvantage of assuming a passive role is that your presence may be considered intrusive. For example, athletes and athletic trainers may be open to your presence in the training room as long as you are involved in various activities. Simply sitting by yourself in the corner of the room with a clipboard makes you conspicuous, and participants may alter their behavior.

If you choose to observe as an active or complete participant, you will have the advantage of fitting in and becoming one of the players in your chosen context. In the previous example of the athletic training room, as a complete participant, you might assist with taping, bandaging, or caring for wounds. Your presence will be less conspicuous, thus helping participants feel more comfortable and freer to be themselves. A disadvantage of this approach is that you must remember the events you observe and document them later. You are limited by the strength of your memory. Your involvement may also be limited by your expertise; don't pretend to know how to tape an ankle just so you can be involved in the setting!

Some researchers strike a good balance with a mixture of both observational roles. In some contexts, you can be part participant and part observer. This approach helps you fit in but still allows you to observe and document your findings when appropriate. Regardless of your method, remember that you are observing a natural setting; your goal is to avoid disrupting it in any way. You must be tactful to fit into the setting, and you must be intuitive to discern when your presence becomes intrusive.

Documents

Qualitative researchers also commonly use documents as data. Examples of documents that researchers may collect in the health profession could include medical records, corporate memos, policy and procedure manuals, court documents, and letters. Although rarely used as primary data, documents often contain information that helps researchers clarify findings from interviews and observations.

Ideally, you will collect data in a variety of ways that inform your interpretation and address your research questions. It would be awesome to have mountains of data at your disposal, but this is rarely the case. Many factors affect your method of data collection, as well as the type and amount of data you choose to collect. Considerations include your time frame, available monetary resources, and access to various contexts and people. You must also consider the strengths and weaknesses of each approach and how each addresses your purpose and research questions.

Once you begin to collect data, you also begin the process of analysis. Remember that you will intuitively begin to analyze even the smallest amount of qualitative data. In fact, the process of data collection and analysis is continuous and ongoing.[34] Qualitative research allows you to analyze your data as you collect it. This differs from quantitative research, in which you first collect all of your data and then analyze it at the end. Over time, you will have a great deal of data to analyze, but the process of analysis is fascinating!

ANALYZING QUALITATIVE DATA

Qualitative data analysis is an interpretive event. In other words, researchers collect and analyze data concurrently and then infer meaning and draw reasonable insights to answer the research questions. Meaning often emerges in a nonlinear fashion as the study progresses during the research process. The analysis process is stepwise and involves specific steps to complete. The most important step in the analysis, however, is becoming familiar with the data. This process is often referred to as being *immersed in the data*, which occurs after reading the transcripts several times and then writing/journaling overall impressions and looking for meaning that will guide the specific steps of the process.

Remember that qualitative researchers attempt to understand the meaning people assign to their experiences. They require an instrument for analysis that is sensitive to speech, writing, and human behaviors to draw conclusions about the qualitative dimension of participants' lives. Therefore, the researcher serves as the instrument for data analysis. From the moment participants share their thoughts, experiences, perspectives, and perceptions, researchers cannot help but wonder what they mean and how they relate to the experience of others.

The process of data analysis requires researchers to use inductive reasoning to categorize information. The process is both creative and structured. We present 8 steps of qualitative analysis based on our research experience and qualitative literature. The process follows the acronym CREATIVE:

Consider your research questions and purpose statement.

Read through your transcripts to gain a global sense of the data.

Examine the data for information related to the research questions and purpose.

Assign labels to these units of information that capture their meaning.

Thematize the data.

Interpret the emergent themes as they relate to the study's purpose and questions.

Verify the findings.

Engage in the writing process to report your findings.

Consider Your Research Questions and Purpose Statement

Revisit your research agenda and carefully review the purpose and the research questions before you begin the analysis process. Simply by doing this you are reminding yourself of the critical information you are seeking. It can help focus and streamline the process. It is important to note, however, to keep an open mind while coding so as not to miss any key or critical information.

Read Through Your Transcripts

Once you have revisited your research questions and purpose statement, you are ready to read your data. Read through your data once without judging the content. This really can be thought of as *preliminary data analysis* and becoming immersed in the data.[35] Immersion can be classified as repeated reading and re-reading interview transcripts and can help provide context and bring clarity to the key findings from the data. The immersion process can make the analysis process more manageable. As you read, make mental or literal notes to yourself about the significance of the content, but try to reserve your judgment until you have examined all of the data.

?

The transcription of my data is 500 pages long. Help!

Welcome to the pros and cons of data collection. The upside is you have lots of good data to choose from, and the downside is that you must work with 500 pages of data! If you read your transcripts as you collect the data, you will be familiar with most of the pages. Remember, you will not use all of the data. Read your transcripts through to get a sense of the whole and direct you to a starting point, which is often not at the beginning!

Examine the Data for Important Information

As you complete the immersion step and gain a better sense of the data, it will be important to highlight, bracket, or tag blocks of the transcripts. This process can include tagging meaningful information that may be a single word, a single sentence, multiple sentences, or a paragraph of text.

Assigning Labels

Labels are assigned to the highlighted, bracketed, or tagged blocks of important information you identified in step 3. These labels are often referred to as *codes*, and the process is often referred to as *coding your data*. Codes are described as illustrative labels that can reflect the meaning of the text and are viewed as the building blocks of the analysis process. Codes are often simply 1 or 2 words used to highlight the overall meaning of that portion of data that has been highlighted.

Thematize the Data

The labeling process, as described earlier, continues during the analysis, as codes begin to be collapsed and organized together to reflect the meaning. The linking or organizing of these codes together is often referenced as *creating categories* or *themes*. Creating categories or themes can be done simultaneously as the labels or codes are assigned. The goal is to create a good fit between the codes that share a relationship. The generation of themes requires interpretation of the codes and labels given previously. This process includes moving beyond basic codes and grouping them to create a category and providing an explanation of the data. A critical step of the thematization process of the data is operationalizing the theme, as well as ensuring it has a relationship to the study's purpose and research questions. It is also important at this time to ensure saturation of the data. Again, this is satisfied when the theme is consistently found among a majority of participants.

? *While examining my data, I realized that 1 piece could be included in 2 different themes. How should I proceed?*

If this happens often and more than 1 piece of data recurs in the 2 themes, consider combining them. You can also place the same piece of data in both themes as long as you clearly justify your decision.

Interpret the Themes

The themes that emerge from your data are your primary findings. You should examine them and interpret the meaning and give them titles that capture their meaning. The title of the theme should relate to the purpose of your study and have relevance for the readers. Moreover, the thematic titles and supporting data should describe the phenomenon or explain the process under investigation. We again use the term *interpret* because our mission with qualitative research is to gain understanding and infer meaning from the data. If your themes do not identify definitive patterns, you have not completed your mission. You must continue to collect and analyze data.

A critical aspect of your data analysis is to consider if and how the emerging themes are related. In many cases, initial themes may be closely related to other themes. Look into any developing relationships that you notice. You may need to combine related themes to clearly capture the meaning of the data.

Data should be collected until you either notice redundant findings or stop discovering new information. We referred to this process earlier as *saturation of data*. When you notice this pattern and can fully answer your research questions, you may conclude the process of data collection and analysis.

Verify the Findings

Although the specific steps to verify your findings are discussed in the next chapter, it is important to briefly mention this as part of the analysis process. Creswell[3] recommends the use of 2 strategies at minimum to verify the findings. Those ways can include member checks, peer review or debriefing, and data triangulation.

Engage in the Writing Process

The next step in the process is sharing the findings after the analysis process is complete. The writing process also allows for critical reflection on the results and findings, and how they are communicated can confirm the emergent data. When presenting the findings it is important to share how the data was coded, but also share with the reader the themes and how they are operationalized, as well as the data used to support the analysis process.

SUMMARY

Rigorous analysis of interview data is an essential aspect of the qualitative paradigm and should be done concurrently with data collection. Each step, however, requires a systematic approach and will require time and effort to complete.

CONTINUE YOUR EDUCATIONAL JOURNEY

LEARN THROUGH ACTIVITY

1. Reflect on the research purpose statement and research questions you created in Chapter 2. Based on this, identify appropriate interview participants and create a semi-structured interview guide.
2. Watch a live event or show on TV, assuming the role of a passive observer. Design, implement, and evaluate an observation instrument that captures the essence of human interactions in the program.

CHECK YOUR KNOWLEDGE

1. While planning a study, you decide that participants should have practiced nursing for at least 15 years. Moreover, these nurses must have some experience with community drug-awareness programs. This scenario represents which of the following sampling strategies?

   a. Chain sampling

   b. Criterion sampling

   c. Maximum variation sampling

   d. Deviant sampling

   e. Typical sampling

2. Over the course of many interviews, you continually hear the same sort of information. Eventually, no new information emerges. Which of the following concepts relates to this scenario?

   a. Triangulation of data

   b. Exhaustion of information

   c. Saturation of data

   d. Redundancy of data

   e. c and d

3. When selecting participants for a study, you purposefully identify only one physician assistant who meets your inclusion criteria, so you decide to rely on this person to connect you with other educators who fit the desired profile. This scenario represents which sampling strategy?

   a. Chain sampling

   b. Criterion sampling

   c. Maximum variation sampling

   d. Deviant sampling

   e. Typical sampling

4. Establishing good rapport with the participant during the initial steps of an interview is known as _____. Speaking to the participant about matters directly related to the research questions is known as _____.

   a. The relational aspect; the thematic aspect

   b. The thematic aspect; the relational aspect

   c. Authenticity; verification

   d. The relational aspect; debriefing

   e. None of the above

5. As part of a research study, you obtain permission to observe an interprofessional education class in a college of health sciences. You are specifically looking to observe interactions among students while working a medical case study. In negotiating your role as observer, you agree to help organize and distribute the materials students will use during their case analysis. Once that task is done, you will simply sit near 2 groups and watch the students. What form of observation does this scenario represent?

    a. Complete participant

    b. Participant observer

    c. Observer participant

    d. Complete observer

    e. Either b or c

6. When analyzing data from a transcript, you identify important information that relates to your research purpose. You then assign this information a label to capture its meaning. This label is also called a _____.

    a. Code

    b. Conceptual label

    c. Meaning unit

    d. Theme

    e. Category

Think About It

1. You interviewed 3 nurses about the key challenges they face in their work environment. When you observe these nurses at work, you notice a substantial difference between what they articulated in the interviews and what occurred at work. Knowing that the process of qualitative research is flexible, how would you proceed?

2. You arranged to speak with a physical therapist as part of a case study, but he has a family emergency at the time of the meeting. How would you deal with this situation?

Make a Stretch

These journal articles will provide further information on the data collection and analysis process:

- Gale NK, Heath G, Cameron E, Rashid S, Redwood S. Using the framework method for the analysis of qualitative data in multi-disciplinary health research. *BMC Med Res Methodol.* 2013;13:117.

- Sutton J, Austin Z. Qualitative research: data collection, analysis, and management. *Can J Hosp Pharm.* 2015;68(3):226-231.

REFERENCES

1. Stringer E. *Action Research in Education.* Upper Saddle River, NJ: Pearson Merrill Prentice Hall; 2004.
2. Patton MQ. *Practical Evaluation.* Newbury Park, CA: Sage; 1990.
3. Creswell JW. *Qualitative Inquiry and Research Design: Choosing Among Five Approaches.* 3rd ed. Washington, DC: Sage; 2013.
4. Palys T. Purposive sampling. In: Given LM, ed. *The Sage Encyclopedia of Qualitative Research Methods.* Vol. 2. Los Angeles, CA: Sage; 2008:697-698.
5. Tuckett A. Qualitative research sampling: the very real complexities. *Nurs Res.* 2004;12(1):47-61.
6. Palinkas LA, Horwitz SM, Green CA, Wisdom JP, Duan N, Hoagwood K. Purposeful sampling for qualitative data collection and analysis in mixed method implementation research. *Adm Policy Ment Health.* 2015;42(5):533-544.
7. Merriam SB. *Qualitative Research and Case Study Applications in Education.* 2nd ed. San Francisco, CA: Jossey-Bass; 1998.
8. Patton MQ. *Qualitative research & evaluation methods.* 3rd ed. Thousand Oaks, CA: Sage; 2002.
9. Bowen GA. Naturalistic inquiry and the saturation concept: a research note. *Qualitative Research.* 2008;8(1):137-152.
10. Morse JM. The significance of saturation. *Qual Health Res.* 1995;5:147-149.
11. Jackson J. A grounded theory of the resilience process in postqualification nursing students. *J Nurse Educ.* 2018;57(6):371-374.
12. Mazerolle SM, Eason CM. Perceptions of National Collegiate Athletic Association Division I female athletic trainers on motherhood and work-life balance: individual- and sociocultural-level factors. *J Athl Train.* 2015;50(8):854-861.
13. Reitz R, Horst K, Davenport M, Klemmetsen S, Clark M. Factors influencing family physician scope of practice: a grounded theory study. *Fam Med.* 2018;50(4):269-274.
14. Mazerolle S, Eason C. A longitudinal examination of work-life balance in the collegiate setting. *J Athl Train.* 2016;51(3):223-232.
15. Petursdottir U, Arnadottir SA, Halldorsdottir S. Facilitators and barriers to exercising among people with osteoarthritis: a phenomenological study. *Phys Ther.* 2012;90(7):1014-1025.
16. Thrasher AB, Walker SE, Hankemeier DA, Mulvihill T. Graduate-assistant athletic trainers' perceptions of the supervisor's role in professional socialization: part II. *J Athl Train.* 2016;51(10):771-779.
17. Flinkman M, Isopahkala-Bouret U, Salantera S. Young registered nurses' intention to leave the profession and professional turnover in early career: a qualitative case study. *ISRN Nurs.* 2013;2013:916061
18. Kvale S. *InterViews: An Introduction to Qualitative Research Interviewing.* Thousand Oaks, CA: Sage; 1996.
19. Schostak J. *Interviewing and Representation in Qualitative Research.* Berkshire, England: Open University Press; 2006.
20. Musselwhite K, Cu L, McGregor L, King KM. The telephone interview is an effective method of data collection in clinical nursing research: a discussion paper. *Int J Nurs Studies.* 2007;44:1064-1070.
21. Cachia M, Millward L. The telephone medium and semi-structured interviews: a complementary fit. *Qualitative Res Organizations Man.* 2011;6(3):265-277.
22. Stephens N. Collecting data from elites and ultra elites: telephone and face-to-face interviews with macroeconomists. *Qualitative Researc.* 2007;7(2):203-216.
23. Sturges JE, Hanrahan KJ. Comparing telephone and face-to-face qualitative interviewing: a research note. *Qualitative Research.* 2004;4(1):107–118.
24. Novick G. Is there a bias against telephone interviews in qualitative research? *Res Nurs Health.* 2008;31(4):391–398.
25. Smith EM. Telephone interviewing in healthcare research: a summary of the evidence. *Nurs Res.* 2005;12(3):32–41.
26. Krueger RA. *Focus Groups: A Practical Guide for Applied Research.* Newbury Park, CA: Sage; 1988.
27. Gill P, Stewart K, Treasure E, Chadwick B. Methods of data collection in qualitative research: interviews and focus groups. *Br Dent J.* 2008;204(6):291-295.
28. Dörnyei Z. Research *methods in applied linguistics: quantitative qualitative, and mixed methodologies.* Oxford, United Kingdom: Oxford University Press; 2007.

29. Kvale S, Brinkmann S. *InterViews: Learning the Craft of Qualitative Research Interviewing.* 2nd ed. Thousand Oaks, CA: Sage; 2009.

30. DeWalt KM, DeWalt BR. *Participant Observation: A Guide for Fieldworker*s. Walnut Creek, CA: AltaMira Press; 2002.

31. Ratner C. Subjectivity and objectivity in qualitative methodology. *Qualitative Social Res.* 2002;3(3):Article 16. doi: 10.17169/fqs-3.3.829

32. Wolcott HF. *The art of fieldwork.* Walnut Creek, CA: AltaMira Press; 2001.

33. Mills GE. *Action research: A guide for the teacher researcher,* 3rd ed. Upper Saddle River: Pearson Merrill Prentice Hall; 2007.

34. Pitney WA, Parker J. Qualitative inquiry in athletic training: principles, possibilities, and promises. *J Athl Train.* 2001;36(2):185-189.

35. Creswell JW. *Educational Research: Planning, Conducting, and Evaluating Quantitative and Qualitative Research.* 2nd ed. Upper Saddle River, NJ: Pearson Merrill Prentice Hall; 2005.

Ensuring Trustworthiness in Qualitative Studies

LEARNING OBJECTIVES

Readers will be able to do the following:
1. Explain trustworthiness in the context of qualitative research and outline the concept's components.
2. Explain strategies for ensuring data trustworthiness.
3. Compare and contrast the concepts of data validity and reliability with data trustworthiness.

It is the researchers' responsibility to convince you to trust their research findings. As a consumer of research, a good approach is to view all research through a lens of healthy skepticism. The quantitative measurement of variables is easily judged by validity and reliability. These traditional terms are not as compatible with the qualitative paradigm because researchers do not attempt to measure variables. However, terms for qualitative research have been developed that closely parallel the quantitative process.[1] Although debate still exists about how to address issues of quality in qualitative studies, the concept of trustworthiness of data and its components of dependability, credibility, and transferability are now standard.[2-4]

VALIDITY

Most scholars consider validity of measures the most important aspect of a quantitative research study.[5] Internal validity, or whether an instrument takes the intended measurement, is an important criterion for psychological variables, like a person's attitude,

Pitney WA, Parker J, Mazerolle Singe S, Potteiger K.
Qualitative Research in the Health Professions (pp 49-58).
© 2020 Taylor & Francis Group.

satisfaction, or agreement in a survey, and physiological variables, like the power of output of a muscle, blood pressure, or blood-lactate levels.

The essence of internal validity is truth and accuracy.[6] From a qualitative perspective, the concept addresses whether the research findings capture what really happened and what participants really meant and believed about a situation. Lincoln and Guba[7] coined the term *credibility*, and many qualitative researchers have since adopted it as parallel understanding of internal validity.[8,9]

External validity relates to how the findings of one study can be applied to other participants or settings. In other words, external validity addresses whether the results of a study can be easily generalized. Qualitative researchers do not usually employ this concept because they are more interested in understanding a specific phenomenon or population. The findings of qualitative research studies are rarely applied to the general population; however, the findings may be applied to similar or related communities. The extent to which qualitative findings apply to other situations is known as *transferability*.

RELIABILITY

Reliability refers to the consistency of measures. Quantitative studies based upon measurements must use an instrument that provides consistent results, regardless of the number of repetitions or amount of rest between trials. To establish reliability, researchers often conduct 2 trials and compare the measured outcomes for similarities. This process is called *test-retest reliability*. Another aspect of reliability is whether results can be reproduced. If a study is repeated using the same procedures, researchers should expect similar results with a small margin of error.

Because qualitative researchers do not rely on measurements and do not perform trials of activities or conduct the same interview twice, they do not worry about whether data can be reproduced. They use the term *dependability* to denote results that are consistent with the data collected.[8]

TRUSTWORTHINESS CONCEPTS

There are 4 overarching concepts of trustworthiness and the equivalent of validity and reliability (credibility, transferability, dependability, and confirmability). Trustworthiness itself is an umbrella term that covers 4 interrelated concepts, including credibility, transferability, dependability, and confirmability. Figure 4-1 provides a brief overview of this concept. In general, researchers can demonstrate their trustworthiness by sharing their backgrounds, qualifications, and experiences. Biographical information can be shared as a means to validate the researcher's viability as a qualified individual to collect, analyze, and share the data.[10] In Chapter 3, strategies were discussed regarding the development of an interview protocol. Trustworthiness can be established when the researcher incorporates iterative questioning (*probes* and *follow-up questions*) into the interview session, which can stimulate greater understanding and remove bias.[11]

Trustworthiness

Credibility	Transferability	Dependability	Confirmability
•Definition: The plausibility of a study's findings •Key question or issue addressed: Do the results capture what is really occurring? •Analogous to: internal validity	•Definition: the ability to apply the findings of a study to similar environments •Key question or issue addressed: is there enough descriptive information to allow a reader to determine whether the results are applicable to similar contexts? •Analogous to: external validity	•Definition: the ability to learn and understand what is really occurring. •Key question or issue addressed: are the results believable? •Analogous to: reliability	•Definition: the findings of a study are neutral in that they are based on data from participants and not a researcher's bias •Key question or issue addressed: are the findings based on the informants' data and steer clear of researcher bias? Analogous to: objectivity

Figure 4-1. Trustworthiness as an umbrella concept.

Credibility

The concept of credibility relates to whether the findings of a study are believable. Some believe that credibility is one of the most critical aspects of trustworthiness. Researchers must take steps to ensure that their findings are accurate and supported by the data. It is the responsibility of the researcher to convince readers that the information he or she presents and reports actually occurred. The details should provide enough support from the standards for credibility. Strategies to address this component of trustworthiness include *triangulation*, *prolonged data collection*, *participant checks*, and *peer reviews*.

How can I be sure that an event described in a report really happened?

Again, qualitative researchers must convince readers that the events they report actually occurred. They should provide enough detail and supporting evidence to meet the standards for credibility.

Triangulation

Triangulation involves using multiple methods, data sources, observers, or theories to gain a more complete understanding of the topic or phenomenon being studied. It can be thought of as a way to cross-check the data. The purpose of triangulation is to demonstrate consistency, not necessarily to yield the same results. Four types of triangulation methods are used to support the credibility of the research study.

Methods triangulation (methodological) is checking the consistency of findings generated by different data collection methods. *Triangulation of sources* is determining the consistency of the data by obtaining data from multiple sources using the same method. For example, Khunti et al[12] examined barriers to healthy lifestyles among students with type 2 diabetes The authors conducted focus groups and observations, while simultaneously administering diet evaluations and questionnaires on physical activity. The triangulation of the methods provided a fuller understanding of the barriers to health perceived by the children. *Multiple analyst* (*analyst triangulation*) uses more than one researcher to analyze and confirm the findings. Different researchers (at least 2) conduct independent analyses and then compare and contrast their findings. Using multiple perspectives or theories to interpret the data is called *theoretical triangulation*. Consider a researcher investigating the educational process in a general education course. This person may choose to interpret the data from a pedagogical perspective and an andragogical perspective, using learning theories from both the adult and child viewpoints.

Triangulation is considered an excellent strategy for ensuring trustworthiness, especially when combined with participant checks (explained next). Table 4-1 summarizes the various methods of triangulation.

Which is a stronger trustworthiness strategy: data-source triangulation or methodological triangulation?

There is no concrete answer to this question. When examining trustworthiness of research, you must consider the entire context of the study.

Prolonged Data Collection

Prolonged data collection (*prolonged engagement*) can yield a deeper understanding, a holistic sense of the research setting, and the assurance that you have captured what really occurred. The idea is that the researcher is able to spend adequate time observing various aspects of the setting or to speak with a range of people to develop a rapport and relationships that offer in-depth insights. Imagine investigating the career experiences of a home health care provider. One interview with the provider and an hour or 2 observing could be very insightful, but it would not likely provide a holistic understanding of the provider's engagement with a patient, interaction with the family, and challenges with acting within a home as compared to a hospital. Prolonged engagement is important, although it does take time, often extending the length of one's study.

Participant Checks

Participant checks, also termed *member checks*, are considered the single most important provision a researcher can make to bolster the credibility of the study.[9,10] There are 2 main ways to complete a participant check: (1) transcript verification and (2) interpretive verification. *Transcript verification* involves the participant reviewing their recorded transcript to ensure its accuracy and content. The process is easy to conduct and includes the researcher sharing the transcript with the participant and asking them for verification and agreement that the transcript matches their intentions. This process should happen prior to data analysis. The *interpretive verification* allows the participant the chance to authenticate the analysis conducted by the researchers. Participants will receive an explanation of the study's findings (often the operational definition of the emergent theme, with supporting data). They will review it and then respond and comment on the viability and plausibility of those findings, as analyzed by the participants.

TABLE 4-1

FORM OF TRIANGULATION

FORM	DESCRIPTION	EXAMPLE	BENEFIT
Data-source triangulation	Researchers obtain multiple forms of data to cross-check information.	They interview stakeholders (eg, teachers, parents, students, business owners) about an issue affecting a school district and community.	Understanding different participants' perceptions helps researchers verify preliminary findings and gain a holistic perspective.
Multiple-analyst triangulation	More than one researcher analyzes the qualitative data.	Three members of a research team analyze interview transcripts and discuss the emerging themes.	Data are examined thoroughly, which ensures that information from participants is interpreted appropriately.
Methodological triangulation	Researchers use more than one method to collect data.	Researchers collect data through interviews, observations, and document analysis.	Researchers verify their findings with a different method, making sure what they observed or recorded in an interview is consistent with what they learned.
Theoretical triangulation	Researchers view the data from different theoretical perspectives.	Researchers analyze data from a study on the perceptions of students with obesity through different lenses: the functionalist perspective and the interactionist perspective.	Different theoretical views of data yield different interpretations. For example, the functionalist perspective finds that environment influences behavior, but the interactionist perspective sees people as active participants in their world.

Even though I have an audio recording of the interview, my participant disagrees with the transcript. What should I do?

1. Return to the recording and check the content again.
2. If you think that the content is clear, play the recording for your participant and articulate your position.
3. Ask why your participant disagrees with the content of the transcript.

If your participant still wants to recant, you must honor that request, even if the information in question is critical to your study.

Peer Review

Peer review is also known as *expert review, peer debrief, independent scientific review,* or *external auditing.*[9] Most often the peer has no connection to the study and has been independent to the data collection or analyses. The peer should have formal training and experience in qualitative research and have content knowledge of the topic under scrutiny. The goal of the peer is to examine both the process in which data are or will be collected and the product of the study (ie, the findings, interpretations, and conclusions are supported by data). The peer review should be focused on 6 components:

1. Background information of the study
2. Data collection procedures
3. Data management procedures
4. Transcripts, field notes, observation summaries, and any other data
5. Data analysis procedures
6. Research findings

The peer review can occur either throughout the study (ie, ongoing) or at the conclusion of the study once analysis has been complete. The review should focus on the six components noted, but can be broken down into stages, rather than done collectively in a retrospective manner.

Who is being debriefed in this process, my peers or me?

You, as the researcher, are being debriefed. Debriefing brings closure to a process or an event. In this situation, you should share what you learned about the process with your peers to the extent that they can verify that what you learned is consistent with the data you collected. This process ensures that your interpretations are appropriate.

The researchers first give the reviewer any background information related to the study's theoretical framework, problem statement, purpose statement, and research questions. The reviewer uses this information to become acquainted with the study's aims and methods to collect and analyze the data. It is important for the researchers to provide details on how they collected data, as well as how it will be analyzed, including a rationale on why it was selected. The peer can become familiar with all aspects of the study without having been a direct part of it. When sharing the results of the study, the peer should be provided with clean transcripts, coded transcripts, field notes, and a schematic of the analysis process. This can include the coding sheet, operational definitions, and the data extracted to support the analyses.

Transferability

Transferability is the ability to extend the findings of one's study to comparable environments or participants. Although results of a qualitative study are not meant to extend beyond its specific parameters, it is possible to demonstrate some applicability to other situations and populations that can be viewed as analogous. Transferability can be compared to external validity of a study using a quantitative paradigm.

Researchers must provide the reader rich, in-depth descriptions on all aspects of the study as a means to provide context and allow the reader to transfer the findings themselves. Transparency is a critical part and should be considered in all aspects of the research report; however, the methods used to analyze the data as well as the findings themselves must be reported in great detail to allow them to be true and, possibly, projected onto other populations and environments.

Dependability

From a qualitative perspective, dependability relates to the research processes that are clear and appropriate. Stringer[13] states that dependability is "achieved through an inquiry audit whereby details of the research process, including the processes for defining the research problem, collecting and analyzing data, and constructing reports are made available to the participants and other audiences." There are close ties between credibility and dependability, and when a researchers ensures one, they often achieve the latter.[9] A peer review, or external audit, often satisfies dependability of a research study.[9] Additionally, providing minutiae of what was done to collect and analyze the data can help satiate the dependability of a qualitative study.

? *If a research study does not address trustworthiness of data, should I read it with skepticism and caution?*

Yes, to a certain extent. The section on trustworthiness often is the first to be cut if a publication is pressed for space. However, a study should include at least one sentence addressing the issue.

Confirmability

Confirmability is to a qualitative researcher as objectivity is to a quantitative researcher. That is, the results must be based on the participants' data, not the biases, preferences, or prejudices of the researcher.[11] Strategies to address this concept of trustworthiness include the previously discuss triangulation and a thorough, rich description of the research methods. In addition to these, an audit trail can be used.

An audit trail is essentially a description of the steps used in the research process, including notes related to one's rationale for the analysis (eg, why coded concepts were grouped or thematized together), as well as a researcher's reflections on the meaning of the data.

SUMMARY

It is important for researchers to implement strategies to ensure trustworthiness of the study. Many viable strategies exist, and Creswell[9] suggests researchers implement 2 at a minimum. Most commonly used are triangulation, participant checks, and peer review. Researchers must describe their study in great detail as a means to establish rigor of the methods and data collected; this includes the strategies selected by the researcher to establish trustworthiness.

CONTINUE YOUR EDUCATIONAL JOURNEY

LEARN THROUGH ACTIVITY

1. Discuss how best to approach participant checks. Would it be best to conduct a participant check via email or in a face-to-face conversation?
2. Examine a qualitative research study and identify the strategy used for ensuring trustworthiness. Explain the extent to which the approach made the results believable.
3. Locate and read 5 qualitative research articles. List the strategies the authors used to ensure trustworthiness and identify which occurred most frequently. Which approach is most commonly used? In your opinion, were these approaches effective?
4. Other concepts related to trustworthiness exist. Search the following terms and create a brief definition of each: (1) authenticity and (2) reflexivity.

CHECK YOUR KNOWLEDGE

1. When an instrument measures the intended variable, it illustrates _____:
   a. Internal validity
   b. External validity
   c. Reliability
   d. Triangulation
   e. a and b
2. The concept of _____ refers to research findings that can be easily generalized.
   a. Internal validity
   b. External validity
   c. Reliability
   d. Triangulation
   e. a and b

3. This concept, a component of trustworthiness, relates to whether a study's findings are plausible.

    a. Validity

    b. Reliability

    c. Credibility

    d. Triangulation

    e. Objectivity

4. This concept, another component of trustworthiness, relates to research processes that are clear and appropriate and have findings that are consistent with the collected data.

    a. Dependability

    b. Transferability

    c. Credibility

    d. Validity

    e. None of the above

5. Which of the following examples is consistent with data-source triangulation?

    a. Two or more analysts examine the data and document their results.

    b. Researchers use different conceptual frameworks as a lens to analyze the data.

    c. Researchers conduct interviews with health educators, parents, and students to understand perceptions of obesity.

    d. Researchers both interview and observe physical educators.

    e. b and c

THINK ABOUT IT

1. You are planning a qualitative research study that examines how physicians maintain balance between work and home. How would you attempt to triangulate your data sources?

2. You show a participant the transcript of her interview as part of your participant checks. She points to a paragraph and states, "I didn't say this. This is not what I said." How would you respond to her? What steps would you take to follow up?

3. You are analyzing data for a study that is using multiple-analyst triangulation. The researchers disagree on the emergent themes. What should the research team do to remedy this issue?

MAKE A STRETCH

These readings will expand your knowledge on trustworthiness of data:

- Elo S, Kääriäinen M, Kanste O, et al. Qualitative content analysis: a focus on trustworthiness. *SAGE Open.* 2014; 1-10. doi: 10.1177/2158244014522633
- Hadi HA, Closs SJ. Ensuring rigour and trustworthiness of qualitative research in clinical pharmacy. *Int J Clin Pharm.* 2016;38(3):641-646.
- Noble H, Smith J. Issues of validity and reliability in qualitative research. *Evid Based Nurse.* 2015;18(2):34-35.

REFERENCES

1. Whittemore R, Chase SK, Mandle CL. Validity in qualitative research. *Qual Health Res.* 2001;11(4):522-537.
2. Sparks AC. Myth 94: qualitative health researchers will agree about validity. *Qualitative Health Res.* 2001;11(4):538-552.
3. Mills GE. *Action Research: A Guide for the Teacher Researcher.* 3rd ed. Upper Saddle River, NJ: Pearson Merrill Prentice Hall; 2007.
4. Guba EG. Criteria for assessing the trustworthiness of naturalistic inquiries. *Educ Communication Tech J.* 1981;29:75-92.
5. Ary D, Cheser Jacobs LC, Razavieh A. *Introduction to Research in Education.* 6th ed. Belmont, CA: Wadsworth; 2002.
6. Silverman D. *Doing Qualitative Research: A Practical Handbook.* Thousand Oaks, CA: Sage; 2000.
7. Lincoln YS, Guba EG. *Naturalistic Inquiry.* Thousand Oaks, CA: Sage; 1985.
8. Merriam SB. *Qualitative Research and Case Study Applications in Education.* 2nd ed. San Francisco, CA: Jossey-Bass; 1998.
9. Creswell JW. *Research Design: Qualitative, Quantitative, and Mixed Methods Approaches.* 2nd ed. Thousand Oaks, CA: Sage; 2003.
10. Patton MQ. Enhancing the quality and credibility of qualitative analysis. *Health Services Res.* 1999;34:1189-1208.
11. Shenton AK. Strategies for ensuring trustworthiness in qualitative research projects. *Educ Info.* 2004;22:63-75.
12. Khunti K, Stone MA, Bankart J, et al. Primary prevention of type-2 diabetes and heart disease: action research in secondary schools serving an ethnically diverse UK population. *J Public Health.* 2007;30(1): 30-37.
13. Stringer E. *Action Research in Education.* Upper Saddle River, NJ: Pearson Merrill Prentice Hall; 2004.

5

Attending to Ethical Issues

LEARNING OBJECTIVES

Readers will be able to do the following:
1. Explain why research is regulated.
2. Identify and explain the principles of research ethics:
   a. Autonomy
   b. Beneficence
   c. Right to privacy
   d. Respect for dignity
   e. Justice
3. Identify the components of informed consent and compose an informed consent form for a qualitative study.
4. Outline strategies for protecting participants.
5. Describe the process used by institutional review boards (IRBs) for approving qualitative studies.

AN OVERVIEW OF RESEARCH ETHICS

Research ethics has received a great deal of attention recently. In response to federal regulations, both universities and private businesses have increased rules for researchers who use human participants. This chapter first explains why research is regulated and identifies the underlying principles of research ethics, including the process of informed consent. It next articulates the role of IRBs in protecting human participants. Finally, it

Pitney WA, Parker J, Mazerolle Singe S, Potteiger K.
Qualitative Research in the Health Professions (pp 59-71).
© 2020 Taylor & Francis Group.

highlights problems that may arise during research and steps researchers must take to protect their participants.

RESEARCH REGULATIONS

Government guidelines, regulations, and requirements are in place because researchers have flagrantly harmed and abused human participants in the past.[1] Examples of these unfortunate historical events include the Tuskegee syphilis study, the Jewish Chronic Disease Hospital study, and the Willowbrook study.[2] Though the specific circumstances differ for each of these studies, they all involve ethical violations of participants, such as intentionally infecting them with diseases, coercing them into a study, failing to inform them of a study's risks, and experimenting on them without their knowledge.

PRINCIPLES OF RESEARCH ETHICS

The theoretical basis of ethics, or moral philosophy, is the foundation of the underlying principles that guide research.[3] Two fundamental theories exist: deontological and teleological ethics. Deontological ethics evaluate the merit of individual actions, regardless of their outcome. For example, if researchers are dishonest to participants about the nature of a study, they violate deontological ethics because honesty is a core value of the research society. Teleological ethics address whether the outcome of a study is good or bad. Does the end justify the means? In the preceding example, the researchers may believe that the outcomes of their study will excuse their dishonest conduct with the participants. Perhaps deceiving participants will lead to remarkable findings and contribute to the good of many people.[3]

? *If I am completely honest with my participants, is there a chance that they will tell me what they think I want to hear?*

This situation is possible. However, if you carefully state the purpose of your study in nonjudgmental terms, your participants should feel comfortable sharing their perspectives.

General principles have emerged from these ethical foundations to guide researchers' actions when developing studies and collecting data from participants. The most common principles were generated by reports of massive abuse, such as the Nuremberg Code from World War II and the Belmont Report from the National Commission for the Protection of Human Subjects of Biomedical and Behavioral Research.[4] The following section elaborates on these general principles:

- Respect for autonomy
- Beneficence (non-malfeasance)
- Dignity and justice

Respect for Autonomy

Researchers protect participants' autonomy by ensuring each voluntarily consents to take part in a study. If participants choose not to be involved, researchers must absolutely respect their decision. Researchers may never threaten people with negative consequences if they do not participate in a study.

Researchers must provide enough information about the study for potential participants to make a rational decision whether or not to be involved.[3] This concept, called *informed consent,* is another element of respect for participant autonomy. Informed consent is often provided in writing.

Composing the Informed Consent Form

The informed consent form explains the following elements of the study:
- The purpose and benefits
- Any possible risks of participation
- Clearly delineated expectations of the participant
- The voluntary nature of participation
- The participant's right to withdraw at any time without prejudice
- How the participant's information will be treated
- The participant's right to ask questions

The informed consent form should be written in plain language (ie, language that is easy for participants to understand). Remember, your participants may not fully understand your subject or theoretical framework. Therefore, it is important to clearly articulate the purpose of your study and what you hope to learn. Explain how the findings of the study will inform current practice or knowledge and benefit others, such as students, teachers, patients, organizations, or professionals. Emphasize that participation is voluntary and that participants can withdraw at any time without consequence. Explain exactly what the participant will do or experience. If you plan to conduct personal interviews, indicate the location, approximate length, and number of interviews. Outline similar details about any intended observations.

(?) *One of my participants withdrew from the study after I collected and analyzed all of the data. Do I need to analyze my entire study again, or can I keep the participant's data?*

Talk to your participant about the situation, but you must respect his or her desire to remove any data.

In the section of the form about treatment of data, explain that you may present or publish your findings in a report. Describe what you plan to do with recordings of interviews and summaries of observations after the study is finished. Finally, you must explain how you plan to maintain the participants' privacy. The main methods of identity protection for participants are anonymity or confidentiality.

Anonymity is rare in qualitative research because it means that researchers do not know the identity of any of the participants. A qualitative researcher could obtain anonymous data from participants by conducting a survey electronically or through the mail. The principle of confidentiality means that researchers know who their participants are but take care to conceal their identities. Qualitative researchers commonly address confidentiality by replacing their participants' names with pseudonyms in transcripts and reports. The informed consent forms with the participants' real names are only seen by the researchers and are locked up safely and never disclosed during or after the study is complete.

Who should create the pseudonyms for my participants and setting?

The pseudonyms must appropriately reflect the culture of the participants and setting, and either you or your participants may select them.

Participants must understand that their questions will be answered. To assist with this, you must provide contact information for members of the research team in case participants have questions about the study itself. If participants have questions about their rights, consider providing contact information for a higher authority, such as a faculty advisor, a school official, the chair of the IRB, or another organizational leader.

The informed consent form is a critical part of qualitative research even if the study poses little or no perceived risk for participants. The use of informed consent is required by federal regulation and is overseen by the Office of Human Research Protections. The Office of Human Research Protections Division of Compliance Oversight reviews institutions' (ie, colleges and universities) procedures for ensuring participants are protected and that ethical principles are not violated. If researchers want to conduct research but they are not associated with a college or university, they are still expected to follow the guidelines from the Declaration of Helsinki that explicates research ethics guidelines. See the "Make a Stretch" section at the end of this chapter for a link to information related to the Declaration of Helsinki.

Participants are required to read and sign the consent form. It is good practice to provide a separate signature line if you plan to record your interviews. Researchers often give participants a copy of the form for their records. Figure 5-1 shows an example of an informed consent form template.

Obtaining Full Consent and Assent

In some studies, it is nearly impossible for researchers to obtain written consent. Other times, consent is implied. In studies based on surveys, researchers use cover letters to explain the study, their expectations of participants, and how they plan to handle returned surveys. Voluntary participation is implied by those who return the survey.

Qualitative researchers who conduct interviews should obtain both written and verbal consent. We recommend asking participants for permission to audio-record the conversation before you start the interview. In a personal interview, begin recording before you ask for permission so you capture the statement of verbal consent if it is given. Turn the device off if the participant does not wish to be recorded. With respect to phone interviews, although the Federal Communication Commission has no rules regarding telephone conversations by individuals, some state laws are in place that prohibit this practice (https://www.fcc.gov/consumers/guides/recording-telephone-conversations).

If you plan to interview minors (people younger than 18 years), you must first obtain consent from their parents or legal guardians. If the legal guardians agree to let their children participate in the study, you must next obtain written assent from the minors themselves.

Name of Sponsoring Institution
Consent to Participate as a Research Subject
Title of Project

Investigators:

Name and Contact Information of Primary Investigators and supervising faculty member (if applicable)

Investigators' Statement

We are asking you to be in a research study. The purpose of this consent form is to give you information you will need to help you decide whether to be in the study or not. Please read the consent form very carefully. You may ask questions about the purpose of the research, what we would ask you to do, the possible risks and benefits, your rights as a volunteer, and anything else about the research or this consent form that is not clear. When we have answered all your questions, you can decide if you want to be in the study or not. This process is called *informed consent*. We will give you a copy of this form for your records.

Purpose of the Study

The purpose of this study is to **(INSERT STUDY PURPOSE)**. **Principle investigator's name** and **title/institution** is conducting the study. You are being asked to participate because **(INSERT SELECTION CRITERIA)**.

Description of the Study

This study will use an exploratory approach to allow the researchers to interview you. The interview will be one-on-one with the researcher and will last about **XX** minutes. You may be asked questions about **(INSERT QUESTION TYPES)**. You may refuse to answer any question at any time.

What is Experimental in This Study?

This is not an experimental study. None of the questions used in this study is experimental in nature. The only experimental aspect of this study is the gathering of information for the purpose of analysis. This investigation will use a series of questions to gather this information. The interview will be tape recorded to help the investigator study the conversation.

Potential Risks

There are minimal risks to you from participation in this study. During the interview, you will be asked to talk about your thoughts about **(INSERT APPROPRIATE DESCRIPTION OF QUESTIONS)**. We do not expect you to experience any discomfort during this study. If you do feel uncomfortable with a question, you do <u>not</u> have to answer that question. If you begin to feel uncomfortable participating in the discussion, you may request to end the interview at any time.

Figure 5-1. Example of an informed consent form template. *(continued)*

Potential Benefits
Describe any potential benefits.

Confidentiality
Participation in this research is voluntary and involves minimal loss of privacy. The interview will be recorded with an audio recorder to help the researcher in the collection of their data. All audio recordings, questionnaires, and data to be used in computer analyses will be assigned an alias or numeric code rather than your own name. **You will be given an alternate name if direct quotes are used in the reporting of the data to protect your identity.** A master list of code numbers will be kept confidential by the researchers and will be stored in a locked file cabinet. All researchers, especially individuals who will code and transcribe the interview sessions, will have extensive training in all confidentiality measures of this study. All other data pertaining to you and other subjects will be kept in a separate locked file in the investigator's office for a maximum period of 7 years. After 7 years, the recording will be erased, and any documents related to the study will be shredded. Confidentiality will be maintained to the extent allowed by law.

Incentives to Participate
The participant will not be paid to participate in this study (**OR DESCRIBE INCENTIVES**).

Costs for Participation
There are no costs associated with participation in this study (**OR DESCRIBE ANY ASSOCIATED COSTS**).

Voluntary Nature of Participation
Participation in this study is voluntary. Your choice of whether or not to participate will not influence your future relations with (**INSERT NAME OF INSTITUTION**). If you decide to participate, you are free to withdraw your consent and to stop your participation at any time without penalty or loss of benefits to which you are allowed.

Questions About This Study
If you have any questions about the research now, please ask. If you have questions later about the research, you may contact **PRINCIPLE INVESTIGATOR** and **CONTACT INFORMATION.**
If you have questions regarding your rights as a human subject and participant in this study, you may call the Institutional Review Board at **SPONSORING INSTITUTION.** The telephone number of the Institutional Review Board is (**XXX) XXX-XXXX.** You may also write to the committee at: Institutional Review Board, **SPONSORING INSTITUTION (email address)** or (**XXX)-XXX-XXXX.**

Figure 5-1 (continued). Example of an informed consent form template. *(continued)*

Consent to Participate

The Institutional Review Board Committee at **SPONSORING INSTITUTION** has approved this consent form as signified by the Committee's stamp. This consent form must be reviewed at least once every year and expires 1 year from the approval date indicated on the stamp.

Subject's Statement

This study has been explained to me. I volunteer to take part in this research. I have had a chance to ask questions. If I have questions later about the research, I can ask one of the researchers listed above. If I have questions about my rights as a research subject, I can call the **SPONSORING INSTITUTION'S** Institutional Review Board Committee at **(XXX) XXX-XXXX.** My signature also indicates that I can change my mind and withdraw my consent to participate at any time without penalty. I will receive a copy of this consent form.

Please initial the appropriate box.

_____   I agree to be audiotaped for study purposes only.

_____   I DO NOT agree to be audiotaped for study purposes only.

_____   _____

Printed name of Participant   Date

_____   _____

Signature of Participant   Date

Figure 5-1 (continued). Example of an informed consent form template.

What should I do if the parent or guardian gives consent but the minor does not want to participate in a study? Similarly, what should I do if a minor wants to participate but the parent or guardian does not consent?

You may not include the minor in your study in either case.

Beneficence

The principle of beneficence, also called *non-malfeasance,* directs researchers to respect the welfare of participants and do no harm. At the very least, researchers must attempt to balance the possible risks of a study with its benefits.[2,3] Forms of risk for participants include psychological, emotional, physical, and social harm.

Richards and Schwartz[5] identify the ways in which qualitative researchers conducting health services research may cause harm. These include anxiety and distress, exploitation by way of power relationships, misrepresentation, identification of participants by others, and inconvenience and opportunity costs.[5] Researchers may cause psychological or emotional harm if the study makes the participants experience stress or anxiety. For example, if you are conducting a study of how athletes cope with the death of a teammate, your interview questions may uncover emotions that the athletes have not processed. They may experience a great deal of stress while discussing their reactions to the death. In instances where stress and anxiety might be predicted, researchers should work ahead to arrange steps for follow-up care.[5]

It is easy to understand how research of professions dealing with health and physical activity may cause physical harm. Tests of physical activity carry inherent risks, as participants may sprain a joint or strain a muscle. Observing a participant's natural behavior, conducting an interview, or examining a participant's written work generates very few physical injuries. Therefore, in most cases qualitative research presents almost no risk of physical harm.

We use the term *social harm* to capture instances where a participant may inadvertently suffer isolation, marginalization, or disaffection due to their involvement in a research study. One way in which this can arise is if you, as a researcher, have a power relationship over someone who is a participant in your study. In such instances there is a risk of harm because if he or she participates in your study, you may learn something about them that causes you to have prejudice against them. Another potential cause of social harm is instances where an informant's identity is not protected. That is, an interviewee's identity is inadvertently made known to others. If an interviewee provided discriminating information about others, he or she may find him- or herself in a difficult situation or predicament. Researchers should take measures to maintain confidentiality of their participants by replacing their names with pseudonyms.

Can I identify my participants to my advisor? If not, how can I demonstrate that I have obtained an adequate pool of participants?

You should be able to explain the range of participants to your advisor without revealing specific names.

Qualitative studies are rarely so sensitive that the process harms the participants, but the potential for injury can be difficult to predict.[2] We recommend you discuss your study with several colleagues or with other researchers who have conducted similar studies to identify any potential risks. Adhering to the principles of beneficence and non-maleficence means you must, as a researcher, consider the balance between the risks of a study and its benefits, and you must clearly indicate the possibility of harm in the informed consent form.[6]

What happens if my study causes an injury to a participant that I had not anticipated? Can I be held liable?

We believe that under tort law you or your institution can be held liable if there is evidence that all 4 of the following components were present: duty, breach of duty, proximate cause, and injury.

Dignity and Justice

As Noble-Adams[2] discussed, the respect of participant dignity relates to not using coercive methods to recruit participants and ensuring that participants are treated in a courteous and respectful manner at all times. Any agreements made between a researcher and participant at the beginning of a study, or at any time during a study, should always be upheld; there is no place for deceptive actions during your research.[7]

The principle of justice, or fairness, requires researchers to treat all participants equitably during the research process. For example, if you advertise an incentive, such as a small gift or gift certificate, for participants who consent to interviews, you must make it available to all the interviewees.

What is the difference between offering an incentive and coercion?

An incentive is usually a small gift or chance to win a small token of appreciation. Coercion is more sinister and suggests a punitive or negative consequence for nonparticipation.

SPECIAL CONSIDERATIONS

Researchers must be aware of special circumstances before beginning a study, such as working with vulnerable participants and identifying situations that may require the disclosure of a participant's involvement and identity.

Respecting Vulnerable Participants

In some studies, you may need to collect data from participants who are part of a population considered vulnerable. Examples include minors (children), prisoners, people confined in detention centers, pregnant people, and people with physical or mental disabilities. Researchers who include vulnerable populations in their studies must take special care to ensure that they do not exploit their participants. Usually, researchers must obtain special permission from the participants' parents, guardians, or administrative supervisors before collecting data.

Disclosing a Participant's Identity

In general, confidentiality dictates the protection of participants' identities. Although extremely rare, some instances necessitate disclosing a participant's identity.

You must disclose the identity of participants who indicate that they intend to harm themselves or others. Consider the previous example of the study about how athletes cope with the death of a teammate. During the course of an interview, a participant begins to cry and states that he can't handle his sorrow. He shares suicidal thoughts with you and threatens to harm himself. Now you must intervene by reporting this information immediately to the appropriate contacts.

You may also disclose a participant's identity in cases of suspected abuse. Consider a study in which you are interviewing children about their physical activity at school and home; you have obtained both parental consent and participant assent to conduct interviews. A child tells you during an interview that her parent strikes her and burns her with cigarettes. You observe bruises on the child's face and burn marks on her arm that support the allegation of abuse. You are now required to act by reporting this information to the appropriate authorities.

You must prepare for these rare instances by understanding your responsibilities and fully inform your participants of actions you may be required to take. Consider adding a statement to your informed consent form that identifies your obligation to intervene, such as, "In case of any threat to yourself or others, your name will be provided to authorities."

INSTITUTIONAL REVIEWS

If you are conducting a study to fulfill requirements for a graduate degree or for future publication, you will probably need to submit your proposal to an IRB. Federal law requires the critical analysis of student proposals by such boards. IRBs pay particular attention to the general principles discussed earlier in this chapter and often require you to complete a form with specific questions like these:

- What is the study's purpose?
- How will you recruit participants?
- What will you require participants to do?
- How will data be collected and managed? Will it be stored in a secure location? Who will have access?
- What are the potential risks of participation in this study? How will you minimize potential harm?
- Will any support services be available to participants?
- What are the proposed benefits of the study?
- Will the study involve members of vulnerable populations? If so, which ones?
- How will you obtain informed consent?
- Have members of the research team had training in research ethics?

In addition to answering these questions, researchers must provide copies of all documents, such as consent forms, cover letters, and interview questions, for review. The IRB panel may ask researchers to clarify or change their procedures if there are undue risks to participants.

As part of the IRB application process, you may also be asked to submit proof of completion of a protection of human subjects research training course. The Collaborative Institute Training Initiative (Human Subjects Research CITI Program) is a widely recognized organization for foundational training in human subjects research. The CITI Program offers specialized content designed for either biomedical or social-behavioral-educational disciplines. Both tracks offer a range of courses designed to educate the researcher on topics such as the historical development of human subject protections, regulatory information, cultural considerations, informed consent, and ethical issues, among others. Human subjects training does not expire; however, refresher courses are available through the CITI Program and are recommended 3 years after initial course completion.

The discussion of research ethics in this chapter relates to the stages of planning, data collection, and data analysis. However, ethical considerations also applies to the process of writing and publishing research. Remember to protect the privacy of your participants in research reports and publications. You must fairly portray the meanings and expressions of your participants when writing your results. Make honest interpretations based on existing data, not data you wish you had collected. Represent your sources accurately and appropriately, giving credit where credit is due.

SUMMARY

Unfortunate historical events generated many research regulations designed to protect human participants from harm. Researchers must be aware of the ethical principles that guide their actions, including respect for autonomy, beneficence, respect for dignity, and justice. Informed consent, usually in writing, is a universal procedure to assist participants to fully understand their involvement in a study and how their data will be treated. The institutional review of research proposals is mandated at colleges and universities and by journal publications to protect human participants and ensure ethical principles are followed.

CONTINUE YOUR EDUCATIONAL JOURNEY

LEARN THROUGH ACTIVITY

1. Find and read 3 published qualitative research studies. Identify potential risks the authors may have considered while conducting their studies.
2. Using the informed consent form template provided in Figure 5-1, design your own informed consent form for a study you are conceptualizing.
3. Ask qualitative researchers how they store transcripts, informed consent forms, audio recordings, and other study materials. Also ask them how they deal with ethical dilemmas during their research studies.

CHECK YOUR KNOWLEDGE

1. Deontological ethics refers to _____. Teleological ethics refers to
   _____.
   a. Whether the outcome of an action is good or bad; whether an action is right or wrong, regardless of the outcome
   b. Whether an action is right or wrong, regardless of the outcome; whether the outcome of an action is good or bad
   c. The culturally sensitive aspects of a social interaction; whether the outcome of an action is good or bad
   d. Whether an action is right or wrong, regardless of the outcome; the culturally sensitive aspects of a social interaction
2. When you ensure that participants voluntarily enter your study, you are following which principle of research ethics?
   a. Respect for autonomy
   b. Beneficence
   c. Justice
   d. Respect for dignity
   e. b and c

3. When you know your participants' names but take measures to conceal their identities, you are following which principle of research ethics?

    a. Disclosure

    b. Autonomy

    c. Anonymity

    d. Confidentiality

    e. c and d

4. Which of the following principles requires researchers to do no harm to participants, or at least to balance potential harm with potential benefits?

    a. Beneficence

    b. Respect for dignity

    c. Non-malfeasance

    d. a and b

    e. a and c

5. Which of the following participant populations are considered vulnerable?

    a. College professors

    b. Students in a juvenile detention center

    c. Patients with Alzheimer's disease

    d. b and c

    e. a and b

THINK ABOUT IT

1. While conducting interviews at a junior high school, a student participant tells you that she has begun to self-inflict wounds to her arms. As you glance at her arms, you see fresh cuts that seem to confirm her comment. What should you do? Who would you contact?

2. A health educator you are interviewing asks you to shut off your recording device and discuss a matter off the record. How would you proceed?

3. You have interviewed and observed a physical therapist for a study. She tells you that she does not have time for the follow-up interview you have scheduled and that she wishes to drop out of the study. What is the most prudent response?

MAKE A STRETCH

The following book and tutorial will expand your knowledge of research ethics:
- Miller T, Birch M, Mauthner M, Jessop J. *Ethics in Qualitative Research*. Thousand Oaks, CA: Sage; 2012.
- The National Institutes of Health's office of extramural research hosts a web-based tutorial for protecting human participants of research studies. Visit the site at http://phrp.nihtraining.com/users/login.php to learn more about research ethics. When you successfully complete the quizzes at the end of the online tutorial, you receive a certificate of completion.
- The *British Medical Journal* has published information about the Declaration of Helsinki. Visit this information at http://www.cirp.org/library/ethics/helsinki/ to learn more about the research principles included in this declaration.

REFERENCES

1. Quinn SC. Ethics in public health research: protecting human subjects: the role of community study. *Am J Public Health*. 2004;94(6):918-22.
2. Noble-Adams R. Ethics and nursing research 1: development, theories, and principles. *British J Nurs*. 1999;8(13):888-892.
3. Aita M, Richer M. Essentials of research ethics for healthcare professionals. *Nurs Health Sciences*. 2005;7:119-125.
4. Jeffers BR. Continuing education in research ethics for the clinical nurse. *J Continuing Educ Nurs*. 2002;33(6):265-269.
5. Richards HM, Schwartz LJ. Ethics of qualitative research: are there special issues for health services research? *Fam Practice*. 2002;19(2):135-139.
6. Houghton CE, Casey D, Shaw D, Murphy K. Ethical challenges in qualitative research: examples from practice. *Nurse Res*. 2010;18(1),15-25.
7. Mills GE. *Action Research: A Guide for the Teacher Researcher*. 3rd ed. Upper Saddle River, NJ: Pearson Merrill Prentice Hall; 2007.

Reporting Your Results and Discussing Your Findings

LEARNING OBJECTIVES

Readers will be able to do the following:

1. Describe participants' demographic information and explain the significance of this process.
2. Describe the structure of a results section.
3. Explain the importance of sharing quotes with a reader.
4. Present quotes that support qualitative research findings.
5. Clarify why pseudonyms are used to present qualitative findings.
6. Identify the influence of a target audience and discipline on the written presentation of a results section.

COMPONENTS OF A RESEARCH REPORT

The term *research report* refers to the outcome of a completed research study. These reports can take many forms, including a thesis, dissertation, published article, or even a technical report to an agency. Regardless of type, the following components should be included in every report:

1. Introduction
2. Review of literature
3. Methods
4. Results
5. Discussion
6. Conclusions

Pitney WA, Parker J, Mazerolle Singe S, Potteiger K.
Qualitative Research in the Health Professions (pp 73-89).
© 2020 Taylor & Francis Group.

Having read the previous chapters, you are probably familiar with the contents of the introduction, literature review, and methods sections. After collecting and analyzing your data, you will be ready to present your results, discuss them, and draw reasonable conclusions.

Chapter 2 outlines the literature review as a separate chapter or section of a proposal. In research reports or journal articles, the literature review is often included as part of an expanded introduction. Some reports require you to share the entire literature review. In these cases, the literature review has its own section that usually appears right after the introduction. Your discipline will determine whether you must include a review of the literature when you submit an article for publication.

When writing a research report, you present your introduction and methods sections in the past tense—that is, in terms of what you have done, not what you will do. Beyond that, the content of these sections is very similar to the proposal. Obviously, you must revise the content to reflect any modifications to your study or procedures. However, because we have already discussed the introduction and methods sections a great deal, this chapter focuses on how to present your results, discussion, and conclusion.

RESULTS SECTION

We now turn our attention to writing the results section of a study. This section first discusses how to consider your audience and how to describe your participants. Next, it explains how to organize your results section to provide an overview of the structure. Finally, it explains how to present the emergent themes, including how to introduce and share quotes with your readers.

Presenting the results of a qualitative study is perhaps the most difficult part of the research process, but it can also be the most enjoyable. You may find this process challenging because you must present a clear, fair, and unobstructed view of others' realities, perceptions, perspectives, and beliefs. You must treat those who have provided you with data justly. You must also be fair to yourself, because you have scoured the data and interpreted the findings. Who knows the relationships among the data better than you?

I know the data better than anyone, but my advisor is disputing my interpretation. What should I do?

First, review your findings to see whether you have adequately presented them. Next, ask your participants to verify your interpretations. Finally, gather your evidence and clearly articulate your case to your advisor. If your advisor still disagrees, call a committee meeting and share your data with others.

In writing your results, you have the opportunity to present your position, explain the evidence you have collected to answer your research questions, help others gain tremendous insights about your investigation, and, most importantly, highlight the voices of your participants. Enjoy this culminating process!

Publication Guidelines

The structure of your report may be significantly influenced by your discipline and the journal in which you hope to publish your work. Reports for dissertations and theses are substantially longer than journal articles. Many journals have size restrictions that limit a report's format. Furthermore, universities often have their own expectations about the format of graduate reports.

You may need to present your report using a specific style that suits your format of publication. For example, if you wish to publish an article in the *Journal of Athletic Training*, you must follow American Medical Association[1] manuscript style. If you wish to publish in *Research Quarterly for Exercise and Sport,* you must follow American Psychological Association[2] requirements. Both styles have instructional manuals that will guide your efforts. Be sure to access them in advance so you can structure your report appropriately.

Participant Descriptions

In your study proposal, you articulated criteria for purposefully selecting your participants. Keep this information in your methods section, but enhance it with new, specific data about your participants that you gathered throughout the course of your study. Present as much descriptive information about your participants as possible to help readers determine the transferability of your findings.

Share the participants' descriptive information, both generally and specifically. First, present demographic information about your participant pool, such as the number of total participants, their average age, the age range, and a breakdown of participants by gender. Other relevant descriptive information includes titles held (eg, department chair, health education faculty, assistant athletic trainer), average years of experience in a particular role, or class standing (eg, senior). Your goal is to carefully craft a description of the group of participants that helps readers understand their background and why they were selected for your study. The following example highlights participant demographic information from a study examining the methods pediatricians use with patients to prevent obesity[3]:

> Pediatricians within the general pediatrics division of the University of Wisconsin provide care to the greater Madison area. Thirty-one spend at least part of their time seeing infants, children and adolescents and therefore were eligible for this study … Together, these physicians have approximately 110,000 patient visits per year … Twenty-four pediatricians (77.4%) were interviewed. They had a mean age of 47 years and had been in practice an average of 17 years at the time of the interview. Forty-two percent were male. Fifty-four percent completed their pediatric residency at the University of Wisconsin and a third practice in private settings.

The authors of this study do a fantastic job situating the context and describing the age, gender, and years of experience of their participants. The authors also provide background information, such as patient visits and geographical location, that is relevant to the study. Readers can use this information to discern how the study's findings might apply to their own situations.

In some studies, I have noticed that researchers refer to their participants as subjects. Is this acceptable terminology?

Many journals are so accustomed to using quantitative terminology that they don't consider using the term *participants*. We believe that the term *participants* is more personal and more accurate because qualitative research does not subject people to interventions or procedures.

You should also share specific information about your participants in a table or other systematic format. Researchers commonly use pseudonyms in place of participants' names when presenting demographic information. The specific information linked to pseudonyms helps readers get to know your participants and relate to their quotes later in the manuscript. You have some flexibility with respect to where you describe your participants. Some journals require you to include this information in the methods section. Other journals view this information as part of your results.

Structuring Your Results

The results section of your study should contain an introductory paragraph, a presentation of the thematic findings supported by quotes, and a conclusion. One way to think of this section is with the old adage, "Let the reader know what you are going to tell them, then tell them what you told them."

The results section of a study may span more than one chapter. Sometimes, especially in dissertations or other large research projects, entire chapters are devoted to individual themes to help readers fully understand the findings. The structure of this chapter reflects the fact that most qualitative publications present the results in a single section. Regardless of how you organize the results section, you must always begin with an introductory paragraph.

Introducing Your Results

The introduction of your results should state both the number of themes that emerged from the findings and their titles. When you use a figure or conceptual model to present your findings, identify it and explain why it provides a good overview. You may need to make a decision about a figure's placement. If a figure only makes sense after a great deal of evidence is presented, it should probably be presented later in the results section.

Introductory paragraphs also outline the rest of the section so readers know what to expect. Consider the following 2 examples of how to introduce result sections. The first example is from the *Journal of Sports Rehabilitation*. Pizzari, McBurney, Taylor, and Feller[4] conducted a qualitative study of rehabilitation programs to identify variables that influenced participants' adherence to the process. At the end of the section on data analysis, they provide a sentence that sets up the first paragraph of the results. We present both the transitional sentence and the paragraph of their results[4]:

Codes were collapsed by grouping together related or similar codes under new headings, and coding was redefined and united until 3 main themes emerged.

Results

The 3 categories of variables identified by participants as influencing rehabilitation adherence were environmental, physical, and psychological factors. Figure 1 shows a flowchart derived from thematic coding of the variables and their thematic groupings.

Here the authors identify the 3 emergent themes and direct the reader to a figure that illustrates their results. Although the authors do not explicitly state what they plan to share with readers, the remaining text uses a subheading to highlight themes so readers can easily understand the content's organization.

The second example is from the journal *Women and Health*. Ball, Salmon, Giles-Corti, and Crawford[5] studied physical activity of women from different socioeconomic backgrounds. Here is how they introduced their results[5]:

Eleven main themes were identified. These were: participation in different types of physical activity, physical activity history, lack of time, planning/routines, lack of motivation, value of sedentary behaviours, social constraints/support, the work environment, local neighbourhood safety and aesthetics, local physical activity facilities, and financial costs of physical activity. The themes are described below.

In this example, the authors clearly articulate the number of themes that emerged from the study. They also explicitly state that they plan to describe each theme. The introduction to your results should lead to the presentation of each theme, which is the most critical aspect of the results section.

Themes

Once you have introduced the findings, you need to present the emergent themes. Use subheadings to organize your content and present the information in a logical manner. You should present and discuss the themes in the order that they appeared in the introductory paragraph.

As you present the emergent themes, remember that simply paraphrasing what you have learned and showing graphics do not convey a depth of understanding and insight. Instead, you must use participants' quotes to support your emergent themes and build a case of truth and believability for your reader.

How much direct evidence should I present to build a believable case?

The quantity of direct quotes depends on your data. You need to find a balance that works for you between the voices of the participants and the researcher.

Researchers commonly present a theme by explaining the meaning of the thematic title and its key aspects. They support the explanation with a direct quote from at least one participant (assuming that they have already conducted interviews). For example, in their 2002 article, Pizzari et al[4] presented the theme of environmental factors in the following manner:

The major environmental factor influencing the completion of home exercise was reported to be lack of time. An abundance of work, holiday, family, and social commitments depleted the amount of time available for rehabilitation. With "just too much (going on) in life" (Belinda), some found that "trying to do rehab around that did get quite difficult" (Mary).

The authors first identified lack of time as a key environmental factor. They then provided short quotes from 2 participants as evidence.

Another important facet of the preceding example is the authors' use of pseudonyms after the participants' quotes. Readers now know that the quotes came from 2 different sources. By sharing quotes from various participants throughout the results section, researchers can give readers a sense of data saturation. If they fail to share pseudonyms in the research report, readers will have no way of knowing whether quotes come from 1 source, 2 sources, or almost all of the participants.

In presenting the emergent themes of a study, researchers must not only explain the findings from their perspective but also clarify the themes by sharing direct quotes from participants. Both practices highlight important issues related to the emphasis researchers place on participants' voices and the way that they present quotes. We begin by discussing the balance between the presentation of researcher and participant voices.

Dominant Voice

When explaining your study's emergent themes and findings, you must decide which participant quotes to use, how many quotes to use, and how much of your voice to share in the results section. These important considerations all relate to the issue of voice emphasis. In other words, which perspective do you wish to emphasize more: the participants', your own, or both equally?

We believe that you must strike a balance between the 2 voices to present the results in a meaningful, compelling, and accurate manner. Having served as the instrument for both data collection and analysis, the researcher (or research team) has listened to participants during interviews, watched their actions, and, in many instances, reviewed numerous related documents. Moreover, the researcher has filtered out unnecessary information, considered important information from many different viewpoints, and cross-checked a great deal of evidence. Who could better explain the emergent findings than the researcher? However, the process of qualitative research is geared toward understanding participants' perceptions of their experiences. The voices of participants highlight the significance of concepts and issues within a given context. From that perspective, who is better equipped to provide a depth of understanding than the participants themselves?

We hope that the preceding paragraph builds a convincing argument for the validity of both voices. Figure 6-1 graphically displays the range of options for balancing voices in the results section. Examples are provided following the discussion of each option. Please note that we do not rank any single method above another. Each method has advantages and disadvantages.

QUADRANT 1: HIGH PRESENTATION OF RESEARCHER'S VOICE; LOW PRESENTATION OF PARTICIPANTS' VOICES. In this method, the researcher's voice is dominant in the explanation of the findings. Subsections of results contain few, if any, quotes from participants and often simply explain the findings from the researcher's perspective. This method is necessary for researchers who consistently hear comments from participants that, however meaningful to the research questions, are extremely pithy.

As an example of this emphasis, we draw from a study by Edmonds[6] who conducted a phenomenology related to nursing students' lived experiences as they engaged in study-abroad programs. Here is an example of high representation of the researcher's voice as Edmonds presented one of her emergent themes[6]:

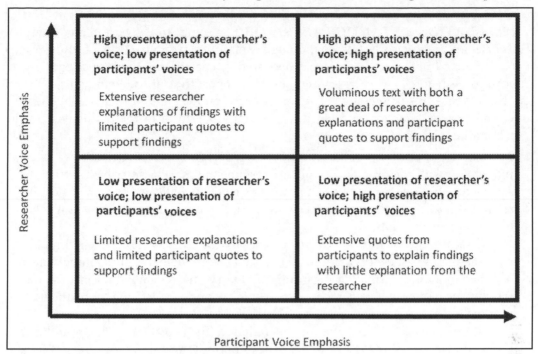

Figure 6-1. Options for voice emphasis.

The second theme that evolved from the data was that of encountering. Within this theme, a strong sense of appreciation was also evident. Encountering was defined as going, doing, and seeing with particular emphasis on the sense of sight. Many participants offered examples of what they witnessed visually during their experience abroad providing evidence that sight was the strongest of the five senses. Encountering reflected the main purpose of study abroad programs, to foster appreciation of the richly contextual array of diverse, sensory experiences one encounters, largely unscheduled, but anticipated. Within this theme, it was discovered that students took advantage of the diverse encounters by actively seeking them out. This finding was somewhat convergent with a theme described by Grant and McKenna (2003) known as "having a go." Their qualitative study findings suggested that Australian nursing students who studied abroad in England and Northern Ireland must display initiative and make the most out of the experience.

Please note that we do not present the entire findings from the theme, but in her study, there are not quotes from participants presented for the theme "encountering." In spite of its lack of quotes, the excerpt fully describes the situation and offers information that supports the emergent category. Researchers may find this method of presenting data useful, but they should not rely on it for entire sections of a report. It is necessary to share participant quotes to enhance the believability of the findings. In the earlier study, Edmonds does indeed present many quotes from students to support the other emergent themes to give readers a rich description of the participants' experiences.

QUADRANT 2: HIGH PRESENTATION OF RESEARCHER'S VOICE; HIGH PRESENTATION OF PARTICIPANTS' VOICES. Some studies have many emergent categories and subcategories. When thorough explanations from participants provide rich details about a finding, researchers may need to fully explain the emergent categories and subcategories before sharing lengthy quotes that support the claims. A study from Pizzari et al[4] illustrates this presentation style. In this excerpt, the authors explain why the type of support a physiotherapist provided to patients was critical to their adherence to the rehabilitation program[4]:

> The most significant part of the rehabilitation process for most participants was their interaction with their physiotherapists. Physiotherapists were described as friendly, knowledgeable, and supportive, and most respondents indicated that their positive relationship with the therapist helped with attending the clinic and completing rehabilitation appointments.
>
> The informational and emotional support provided by physiotherapists throughout rehabilitation was important to all participants. Particularly in the initial stages of rehabilitation, information regarding the injury and rehabilitation process was thought to be vital for adherence. When information was lacking, nonadherence resulted.
>
> "I started physio 3 weeks after my operation…. The people at the hospital didn't really inform me of what I had to do. I mean maybe it was naïve to think I'd get a phone call to say 'You have to start physio,' but I suppose that's what I was thinking at the time. I wish I'd have known and I would have started it earlier. I mean, I knew I had that sheet from the hospital, on 2 separate occasions, and I wish they'd have stressed more that the first couple of weeks was the most important, just to keep it moving, because I don't think I moved it enough. And I think that … took me longer to get started. So, the first couple of weeks of physio was sort of like behind" (Belinda).

As you can see, the authors begin with their own interpretation of the findings and then support it with a long participant quote. This presentation style offers a comprehensive picture and fully describes the findings.

QUADRANT 3: LOW PRESENTATION OF RESEARCHER'S VOICE; LOW PRESENTATION OF PARTICIPANTS' VOICES. In some instances, the presentation of qualitative findings highlights neither the researcher's voice nor the participants' voices. This situation is rare, but writers are sometimes forced to use this presentation style by a journal's space limitations. Consider the following example from a study about participants with multiple sclerosis who completed a resistance-exercise program.[7] The authors presented data within the theme of "positive physical outcomes." Here is the introduction of the theme:

> Not unexpectedly, all nine participants reported that they felt stronger at the end of the program. Four participants noted improved endurance and two participants noted improved flexibility: participant 1 "noticed more dexterity in my fingers," while participant 6 observed "less stiffness…. I always used to feel stiff."
>
> Five participants also reported that various activities of daily living had improved. Participant 2 stated that with walking "I used to stagger, trip … and since I've been doing strengthening I've noticed it a lot less." Participant 6 felt that "walking up a set of stairs with shopping doesn't seem to concern me too much anymore."

As you can see, the authors neither provide lengthy quotes from participants nor offer an exhaustive interpretation. However, the authors also explain their findings with a visual diagram. We would like to note that this style of emphasis works well within the context of this particular study. The authors did not need elaborate explanations to convey their findings.

QUADRANT 4: LOW PRESENTATION OF RESEARCHER'S VOICE; HIGH PRESENTATION OF PARTICIPANTS' VOICES. Some authors prefer to stay out of their presentation of the findings. Instead, they use extremely long quotes from participants in the results section and offer very little interpretation. Researchers commonly use this approach in narrative studies, which focuses on the life stories.

This presentation style is also rare and is not compatible with the space limitations of journal publications. Theses and dissertations have fewer space requirements, so authors have more freedom to use lengthy participant quotes. Consider the following example that emphasizes participants' voices[8]:

Emotional Support

According to many of those interviewed, emotional support was the number one type of support needed by an injured athlete. One coach said "The greatest need of an injured athlete is emotional support … making sure that emotions are getting taken care of." Another coach advised "… be consistent with injury as with other psychological issues with athletes." An athletic trainer agreed by saying "The mind is very powerful and controls everything in the body.… It is important to support them emotionally in order to keep their mind focused on the task of rehab." Another athletic trainer said "It is all about emotions when injured." One athlete said "Emotional support is most important because when injured emotions are going all over the place.… You need people to keep you going."

Another form of emotional support is that of encouragement. One athlete believed "… encouragement, that's what it is all about." Other injured athletes agreed by saying "Knowing people are behind you.… Encouragement and reinforcement are great," "Real positive encouragement is needed and helped me … see the brighter side of things," and "Encouragement from coach really helped me, emotionally and all."

Coaches also realized the need for encouragement saying "… me supporting them and encouraging them is very helpful emotionally" and "… encourage the injured athlete … it is hard work to heal and get back to playing." One athletic trainer said "My job has a lot of different responsibilities.… I need to work with the body to heal and recover, but it is also my job to encourage them [injured athletes], encourage them in healing and encourage them in their mindset.… Not all athletes feel the same way about injury, but [it] is important to make sure they feel encouraged and are emotionally stable … there are many emotions present when an athlete gets injured, part of my job is to deal with those."

Yet another important component of emotional support is understanding. Athletes commented "The athletic trainer had an understanding of the situation" and "Coach understands and works with me." One athletic trainer also recognized the importance of the coach understanding in stating "It is important for the athlete to have understanding from the coach." When talking about support given to injured athletes, one coach said "The coach and athletic trainer need to respond well to injury and understand the athlete might have a wide variety of feelings at first."

Consider these 4 styles when presenting your data. Hold your readers' interest by varying your emphasis of voices. We suggest that you borrow techniques from each quadrant as you present your results. The next section provides suggestions about presenting your quotes.

Quotes as Evidence

In presenting your themes, you must share participant quotes. The quotes are the raw data that informed your coded concepts in the first place, which were then used to form your themes. Use them to bring your results section to life and help readers make clear links between the quotes and the themes.

Quotes can be presented in many ways. You can use long, block quotes; quotes of medium length that are integrated directly into a sentence; or very short, pithy quotes. This section explains each type of quote. As you read it, keep your audience in mind. Remember that your readers will appreciate a variety of presentation. Therefore, we recommend using quotes of different lengths from various participants. Compare this practice to sentence structure. If every sentence in a paper were complex, readers would soon lose interest. You also need to use simple sentences. A combination of simple and complex sentences creates a unique rhythm and makes the text easy to read. Participants' quotes can achieve the same balance.

USE BLOCK QUOTES. Long participant quotes give readers a rich sense of context and almost allow them into the minds of participants. Consider Pizzari and colleagues'[4] explanation of how time restraints affected their adherence to rehabilitation:

> Being a mother ... you have to prioritize and you get to be good at doing that you know, so you sort of like think "I've got to do this, I've got to do that," and in your mind you're already thinking "I've planned this and planned that," and we can do it you know ... you just prioritize what you need to do and get the job done (Jane).

INTEGRATE QUOTES INTO A SENTENCE. Sometimes a short, concise quote adequately conveys meaning and offers evidence for a claim. Short quotes can be worked right into the body of a sentence. For example, in a study on disability and the mediating effects of physical activity, Goodwin, Thurmeier, and Gustafson[9] presented a theme titled "Don't treat me differently" and explained how one participant described a normalizing experience. Here is how the authors integrated a quote into the body of a sentence:

> Although not all of the participants drove cars, those who did spoke of what a normalizing experience it was. Fellow drivers were unaware of the participants' impairments thereby eliminating the dependency assumption. Liz recollected, "I'm hollered and honked at just as much as anyone; I get the same treatment. I love driving because when I'm driving I'm just me and nobody has any reason to believe I'm not like any other driver."

USE PITHY QUOTES. Sometimes, no matter how many ways you ask a question, participants simply do not give an elaborate response. Qualitative researchers who primarily interview teenagers often encounter this problem. Don't fret if your evidence mostly consists of very short comments. You can still use these quotes. In fact, the presentation style from quadrant 3 is very appropriate for short, pithy quotes. Remember that you can only work with the data you have obtained, so you must do the best you can.

We refer back to the work of Dodd et al[7] because they did a good job of using and presenting pithy quotes. Another theme they presented was related to the positive social outcomes patients with multiple sclerosis experienced by participating in resistance-training programs.

The authors weave and integrate quotes from several different participants into their sentences:

> The eight participants who completed the programme valued the social aspect of the programme, including the companionship and friendships that developed. Participant 2 stated that she had "formed new friendships," participant 8 "loved the atmosphere … the group was nice," and participant 6 "enjoyed everybody's company … the camaraderie."

You have many options when presenting your evidence. Remember to vary your use of quotes, as well as the length of your own commentary. From a reader's standpoint, the results will flow much better and make the reading process more enjoyable.

When I integrate participants' quotes into my research report, should I correct their grammar?

You must maintain the integrity of the meaning that the participant provides and be sensitive to their verbal and cultural expressions. However, you must also ensure that readers will understand the quotes and their connection to the theme. Occasionally, you may need to remove extraneous utterances like "um" or add a clarifying term or phrase in brackets.

Summary of Results

Once you have presented your emergent themes, you must summarize them. When a results section has many themes, lots of quotes, and rich information, you should provide a paraphrased summary. This section gives you one last chance to concisely state the thematic findings; however, summaries are not required. Many published studies omit this part of the results section because of space limitations. Another reason a summary may be omitted is that the discussion section of a manuscript often restates the study's purpose and findings.

DISCUSSION SECTION

In a research report, the discussion should present a thoughtful discourse that links your findings with relevant literature. It should follow a coherent introductory paragraph with a systematic presentation of findings that are situated within the context of the literature. The discussion concludes by presenting any implications the findings present for theory, practice, or policy.

Introducing the Discussion

The introductory paragraph should restate the purpose of the study and then provide a general statement about its findings that reminds readers of the context. Although this practice may seem a little redundant, remember that some readers skip straight to the discussion section to discern the essence of a study. When introducing your discussion, remember to revisit your purpose statement and research questions. If you fail to do this, the readers may feel a bit cheated. Consider this example from a study from Mazerolle, Gerhard, and Eason,[10] who sought to explore the work-life balance perspective of athletic trainers who were employed at institutions of higher education that used a medical model approach to delivering health care to intercollegiate athletes:

> After the initial analysis of data, three dominant themes emerged: role congruity, work time control, and collegial relationships (Table 2). The separation of the athletic training department from the athletics department became a noticeable sub-theme within the area of role congruity. Similarly, professional commitment appeared to be a sub-theme of collegial relationships. Each of these sub-themes are presented with supporting [participant] quotes.

? How many times should I present the purpose of my study?

In an ideal world, all readers would view our work in the order we wrote it. However, just as you may have jumped around while reading this book, students may elect to read your work in the order that makes sense to them. Therefore, you should reiterate the purpose statement at the beginning of a discussion. In a thesis or dissertation, expect to restate the purpose statement at the beginning of each chapter. Don't fight it, just do it!

Body of Text

When writing the body of the discussion, be sure to systematically discuss your findings in the same order that you presented them in the results section. This practice adds logic and order to your overall presentation. When discussing your findings, you have some freedom to speculate about the meaning of the findings, but readers will expect you to compare and contrast your findings with existing literature.

You have 2 options for relating your study to existing literature. You can first discuss the finding itself and then explain the relationship. Your other option is to discuss the literature before articulating your findings. We present examples of each technique. The first example presents the finding from the study first. The second example leads with a literature citation. Both methods of presentation are appropriate.

? I know I need to link my results to the literature in the discussion section. Can I introduce new literature at this point, or should I only refer to literature included in the review?

Again, it depends on your intent. Are you introducing new literature because your findings led you down a different path or because you simply missed these articles in your literature review? The former might be anticipated, but the latter is unacceptable.

In a study of women with disabilities and their perceptions about aging, Goodwin and Compton[11] relate the loss of physical freedom, one of the findings from their study, with 2 sources from the literature:

> The potential for decreased independence with age elicited strong psychological feelings about the women's quality of life. The women were disheartened about the

prospect of requiring the assistance of others. A depressed mood state has the potential to negatively impact the incentive needed for the women to continue to be causal agents in their own health and physical well-being and maintain physical function as long as possible. (Dunn, Trivedi, & O'Neal, 2001; Moore et al., 1999) (p. 135)

In a study of the professional socialization of athletic trainers who work in the intercollegiate setting, Pitney[12] related findings in the literature with those in his study:

Bureaucratic influences have the propensity to create routinization of work and managerial control, increase volume of work, and down-grade job-related tasks and skill levels. The participants experienced several of these aspects, including increased work volume, impersonality (lack of support and appreciation by administration), and hierarchy of authority.

Results that are noteworthy and very unique require discussion, regardless of whether comparable literature exists. Hodge, Tannehill, and Kluge[13] used this tactic in discussing a noteworthy finding:

In addition to the teaching variables listed above, and not surprising, journal entries included reference to organization and class management. They reflected on the importance of establishing rules and routines as helping to manage the youngsters' behaviors. Moreover, students pointed out that social reinforcement (eg, verbal praise), token economy system, and physical activity reinforcers following Premack principles were useful strategies for managing youngsters' behaviors. Further, they reflected on the humanistic, educational, and social values of inclusive physical activity programming.

Even though the preceding paragraph does not articulate a relationship to other sources, the authors discuss informative findings that may help readers, particularly educators, understand how the journaling process identifies helpful strategies for class management.

Limitations

No study is perfect! Acknowledge your study's limitations. In other words, every study has at least one drawback. You have an obligation to share them with readers. For example, one key limitation of qualitative research is that the results cannot be generalized for a vast population. When you write a research report, consider placing your limitations at the end of the discussion section, before you conclude your study. This practice is different from a proposal, which shares potential limitations in its introduction.

Conclusions and Implications

End your report with conclusions, implications, or a combination of both. The conclusion should provide answers to your research questions and summarize the study's findings. You can also identify practical implications that your study generated. Try to add a new level of significance for your findings, and point out practical solutions for any identified problems.[14]

The conclusion section commonly includes suggestions for future research. For example, Hodge et al[13] wrote, "To learn more about how to guide students in the journaling process, future research could focus on the experience of journaling as a form of self-reflection." This is an excellent place for novice researchers to obtain ideas for their own projects. As another example, Mazerolle and colleagues[10] offered this in their implications section:

> The current findings continue to illustrate the importance of a supervisor who is an advocate for his or her employees and continues to them professional and personally. Autonomy and job flexibility were provided to our participants, and this was directly attributed to the management and leadership of the head athletic trainer.

Also in this section of a paper, many authors present implications for future research. For example, after presenting the findings and a conceptual model regarding clinical decision making in acute care physical therapy practice settings, Masley, Havrilko, Mahnensmith, Aubert, and Jette[13] added the following to comment on directions for future research:

> Our model needs to be validated with different groups of physical therapists in the acute care setting because models of practice and roles of physical therapists may vary in different parts of the United States and around the world. Additional areas of research that could be explored include a comparison of clinical reasoning processes and decision making across physical therapy settings. Future research could also include an investigation of why physical therapists choose different settings in which to practice, illuminating key skills and personality traits that may be more suited to one type of practice environment than another and helping students and novices evaluate their career options.

FINAL REVIEW

Once you have completed your results and discussion sections, you should revisit your title and modify it, if necessary. Many journals prefer a title to capture the study's conclusions. Remember that the title will help others locate your study. It should succinctly capture the content of your study, but be general enough that readers will be able to access it with a research database or search engine.

You must also create an abstract that provides a concise (usually no more than 400 words) summary of your study. The abstract should include information related to the study's objective; design; participants; methods of data collection; and analysis, results, and conclusions. Most journals also require you to include key words at the end of your abstract. The key words should differ from those in the article's title.

(?) *Does the title really matter?*

Yes! The title is important because it is the first part of the study your readers will see. You must strike a balance between catchiness and content. The title must pique the readers' interest but be easy to locate with current research databases. Conduct a search using common descriptive terms for literature on your topic. Ask yourself whether you would be able to find your own study if you were to redo your literature review.

As you assemble your manuscript, visit the authors' guide for information about the order of the materials and how to display various items. For example, you may be required to present all of your figures at the end of the manuscript, rather than within the body of the text. Every journal operates differently, so be aware of the specific guidelines.

SUMMARY

The results section of a well-written qualitative study uses quotes to support emergent themes. As authors interpret the findings and paraphrase the data, they must provide participant quotes that support the claims and substantiate the findings. They should share quotes in a variety of ways to make the report easier to read.

In the discussion section, authors should first remind readers of the study's purpose, then compare and contrast the findings with related literature. They should draw reasonable conclusions and identify implications for future research based on the study's results.

CONTINUE YOUR EDUCATIONAL JOURNEY

LEARN THROUGH ACTIVITY

1. Select a published qualitative research study and examine the results section for descriptions of participants. How many people participated in the study? What were their ages, genders, and ethnicities?
2. Evaluate the authors' use of participant quotes. In which quadrant did they present the majority of evidence?
3. Read the entire article and write a 400-word abstract. Please challenge yourself and do not use aspects of the abstract provided.
4. Identify the limitations of the study described by the authors. What other limitations can you identify?

CHECK YOUR KNOWLEDGE

1. The structure your report takes may be significantly influenced by your _____ and the _____ in which you hope to publish.
   a. Research budget; website
   b. Discipline; journal
   c. Writing ability; website
   d. Research budget; journal

2. It is critical to describe your participants, but you must also protect their identities. Which of the following is an acceptable way to protect the identities of research participants?
   a. Never use their quotes.
   b. Always provide their real names.
   c. Use pseudonyms.
   d. Consider using only sources that allow you to publish their names.
   e. b and c

3. How can you use quotes to support your research findings?
   a. Use block quotes.
   b. Work your quotes into the structure of the sentences.
   c. Present the data by paraphrasing its meaning.
   d. a and b
   e. All of the above are useful ways to present research findings.

4. When writing a discussion section, it is not important to utilize existing literature.
   a. True
   b. False

5. Which of the following is true of the discussion section of a research report?
   a. You should remind the reader of your study's purpose.
   b. You should compare your research findings with those in existing literature.
   c. You should contrast your research findings with those in existing literature.
   d. b and c
   e. a and b
   f. a, b, and c

THINK ABOUT IT

1. In your opinion, what is the most important aspect of a discussion section?
2. Why should authors provide practical suggestions about the implications of a study?
3. What ethical obligations do researchers have while presenting the findings of a study?
4. When presenting quotes, some researchers use pseudonyms and others use participant numbers in place of names. Identify the advantages of each method.
5. One of your participants is not a native English speaker. The transcript of the conversation is very fragmented. How might this affect your presentation of the results?

MAKE A STRETCH

These readings will expand your scholarly communication skills.

- Knight KL, Ingersoll CD. Optimizing scholarly communications: 30 tips for writing clearly. *J Athl Train.* 1996;31:209-213.
- O'Brien BC, Harris IB, Beckman TJ, Reed DA, Cook DA. Standards for reporting qualitative research: a synthesis of recommendations. *Acad Med.* 2014;89(9):1-7.
- Tong A, Sainsbury P, Craig J. Consolidated Criteria for Reporting Qualitative Research (COREQ): a 32-item checklist for interviews and focus groups. *Int J Qual Health Care.* 2007;19:349-357.

REFERENCES

1. American Medical Association. *Manual of style: A guide for authors and editors.* 10th ed. New York, NY: Oxford University Press; 2007.
2. American Psychological Association. *Publication manual of the American Psychological Association.* 6th ed. Washington, DC: American Psychological Association; 2010.
3. Gilbert MJ, Fleming MF. Pediatricians' approach to obesity prevention counseling with their patients. *Wisconsin Med J.* 2006;105(5):26-31.
4. Pizzari T, McBurney H, Taylor NF, Feller JA. Adherence to anterior cruciate ligament rehabilitation: a qualitative analysis. *J Sport Rehab.* 2002;1190-102.
5. Ball K, Salmon J, Giles-Corti B, Crawford, D. How can socio-economic differences in physical activity among women be explained? A qualitative study. *Women Health.* 2006;43(1):93-113.
6. Edmonds JL. The lived experience of nursing students who study abroad: a qualitative study. *J Studies International Educ.* 2010;14(5):545-568.
7. Dodd KJ, Taylor NF, Denisenko S, Prasad D. A qualitative analysis of a progressive resistance exercise programme for people with multiple sclerosis. *Disability Rehab.* 2006;28(18):1127-1134.
8. Borseth KM. An *Investigation of the Social Support Network of Injured Athletes* [unpublished master's thesis]. De Kalb, IL: Northern Illinois University; 2004.
9. Goodwin DL, Thurmeier R, Gustafson P. Reactions to the metaphors of disability: the mediating effects of physical activity. *Adapted Phys Activity Quar.* 2004;21:379-398.
10. Mazerolle SM, Gerhart ST, Eason CM. Exploring the effect of the medical model organizational structure on collegiate athletic trainers' quality of life: a case study. *Athl Train Sports Health Care.* 2018;10(4):159-168.
11. Goodwin DL, Compton SG. Physical activity experiences of women aging with disabilities. *Adapted Phys Activity Quart.* 2004;21:122-138.
12. Pitney WA. Organizational influences and quality-of-life issues during the professional socialization of certified athletic trainers working in the National Collegiate Athletic Association Division I setting. *J Athl Train.* 2006;41(2):189-194.
13. Hodge SR, Tannehill D, Kluge MA. Exploring the meaning of practicum experiences for PETE students. *Adapted Phys Activity Quart.* 2003;20:381-399.
14. Booth WC, Colomb, GC, Williams JM. *The Craft of Research.* 2nd ed. Chicago, IL: University of Chicago; 2003.

PART THREE

Advanced Concepts of Qualitative Research

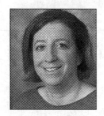

Qualitative Research in Medicine

I do not remember any discussion of qualitative research during medical school and very little mention of qualitative methods during my residency training. My professors taught us how to evaluate quantitative research and understand statistical tests, however, no qualitative studies were introduced during journal clubs or presented as evidence for how to care for patients during my medical education. When I began practice as a sports medicine physician, I felt that my understanding of how to design, carry out, and interpret research was incomplete, and I decided to pursue a master's degree in clinical investigation. The first class I signed up for was an introductory class on qualitative research, because its concepts were the most foreign to me. The class exemplified the phrase "you don't know what you don't know" and helped give me a sense of the complexities of qualitative research. I learned that for my next research study on concussion education in youth sports, I should include an investigator with an understanding of qualitative research that was much deeper than my own.

My interest in qualitative methods is linked to my interest in how research benefits individuals at the community level. What good is research if its results are not tied to improved health outcomes at the individual level? I work at an elite academic medical institution, the type of organization where the importance of research dissemination can get lost. I am not just interested in the propagation of information from academics to patients. I believe that community members and organizations deserve the opportunity to help form research questions and participate in the design of projects that involve them (ie, community-based participatory research).

While a randomized controlled trial may be the best method to assess the efficacy of a new cholesterol medication, a study with focus groups may be more effective to determine parents' concerns about sports injuries during football games. Quantitative methods, such as interviews, focus groups, and observation, allow a unique type of input from individuals.

There is still a lack of understanding about how qualitative research methods can answer questions that quantitative approaches cannot. While I was presenting focus group data from our study involving parents of youth football players at a national conference, I heard a colleague say "So that's what counts as research now? Sitting around talking to a bunch of parents?" However, there are some questions that quantitative methods cannot answer. The themes that arose from our focus group study led us to develop educational materials about the sports concussion prevention that addressed the concerns voiced by community members. The qualitative data also complemented quantitative survey data we obtained.

About Dr. Carl

Dr. Carl is a graduate of the University of Illinois College of Medicine. She completed her residency in pediatrics at the University of Wisconsin Hospital and Clinics. She completed a fellowship in primary care sports medicine at Rush University Medical Center and a fellowship in nonoperative pediatric orthopedics at the University of Wisconsin Hospital and Clinics. Her specialty is in primary care sports medicine and nonoperative orthopedics and her clinical interests include scoliosis, gait abnormalities, developmental orthopedics, hip dysplasia, sports-related concussion, sports injuries, and injury prevention. Her research interests include injury prevention, youth participation in boxing/martial arts, and clubfoot.

Rebecca Carl, MD

Attending Physician, Institute for Sports Medicine
Ann & Robert H. Lurie Children's Hospital of Chicago
Assistant Professor of Pediatrics
Northwestern Feinberg School of Medicine
Chicago, Illinois

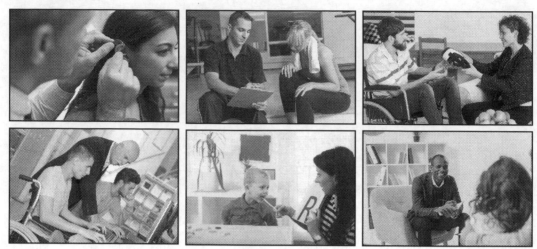

Part Three begins with Chapter 7, which presents specific forms of qualitative research. This chapter focuses primarily on grounded theory, ethnography, and phenomenology but also presents qualitative case studies, narrative inquiry, and action research. Chapter 8 presents information on mixed methods research—a common research approach in the health professions.

Chapters 9 and 10 pertain to how to gauge the worth and merit of qualitative research. First, Chapter 9 provides several frameworks for evaluating a published qualitative study. Chapter 10 addresses the role that qualitative research plays in evidence-based practice. Evidence-based practice is a mainstay in health care interventions but has had a focus on the use of quantitative information. We present perspectives that will display how qualitative research can be used as evidence. Additionally, we will explain how qualitative methods can help practitioners contextualize evidence and determine how context may influence the use of evidence.

Our final chapter examines the most common arguments and assumptions made against qualitative research and offers suggestions on how to respond to critics. Chapter 11 also presents practical advice and resources for continuing your journey as a qualitative researcher.

GUIDING QUESTIONS

Consider the following questions before reading Part Three. They will guide your examination of each chapter.

1. What forms of qualitative research exist? How are they similar to and different from one another?
2. In what ways do qualitative and quantitative studies complement one another?
3. How can a research study combine qualitative and quantitative methods to address its purpose?
4. When is it appropriate to design a study that includes both qualitative and quantitative methods?
5. What is evidence-based practice, and how is qualitative evidence used in this process?
6. What factors should you consider when evaluating a qualitative research study?
7. How does your purpose for evaluating a study influence the questions that you ask?
8. What are common criticisms of qualitative research?

7

Understanding Forms of Qualitative Research

LEARNING OBJECTIVES

Readers will be able to do the following:
1. Identify various forms of qualitative research.
2. Explain the focus of grounded theory, phenomenology, and ethnographic studies.
3. Compare and contrast methods of data collection and analysis used with grounded theory, phenomenology, and ethnographic studies.
4. Describe research products associated with the forms of qualitative inquiry.

BEYOND THE BASICS

The preceding chapters introduced the basic, generic approach to qualitative research. We borrow the term *generic* from Merriam,[1] who articulates that this is indeed the most popular way to conduct qualitative research. The premise of our text was that the way in which data are collected and analyzed is similar, regardless of the form of qualitative study that is performed. Thus far you have learned the basics of inductive analysis that is transferable to all forms of qualitative inquiry. A basic approach to qualitative research is a very pragmatic way to approach the research process.

However, if you want to learn more about qualitative research and to conduct future studies, you should know that many forms of qualitative research exist. In order to be an educated consumer and astute researcher, you must be able to recognize the various forms of inquiry and understand the focus, method, and product of each.

The differences between the forms of qualitative inquiry are quite interesting. We believe Schram[2] said it best with the following quote: "[w]ays of looking—observing,

Pitney WA, Parker J, Mazerolle Singe S, Potteiger K.
Qualitative Research in the Health Professions (pp 93-107).
© 2020 Taylor & Francis Group.

asking, and examining what others have done—are notably similar across many qualitative research traditions. Ways of seeing—encompassing underlying intent, guiding concerns, focus, and perspective—are not so similar."

As we explore the common forms of qualitative research, keep in mind that no one way of examining the social world of others is most correct.[3] Indeed, there is a great deal to consider when choosing an approach. The form of qualitative research that you choose depends not only on the purpose of your study and research questions but also on your philosophical stance and personality.[3] This chapter, therefore, introduces various forms of qualitative research, including grounded theory, ethnography, and phenomenology. It discusses the focus, method, and product of each form and lists examples of research purposes and questions for each. The chapter concludes with a small section on forms that are less common, including qualitative case studies, action research, and narrative inquiry.

GROUNDED THEORY

Grounded theory is an approach to qualitative research that originated in the Chicago School of Sociology between the 1920s and 1950s.[4] Two American sociology researchers, Glaser and Strauss, are credited with bringing direct attention to this method of inquiry. In the 1960s they created a very systematic way to analyze qualitative data and generate theory.[5]

The initial process for developing grounded theory was termed the *constant comparison method*.[6] It is composed of the following distinct stages:

1. Identifying and comparing information or incidents
2. Developing categories and constructing subcategories
3. Delimiting the theory
4. Explaining the theory

These stages, although still used in many qualitative studies today, have been refined. In fact, grounded theory has evolved considerably since the 1960s, largely due to the work of Glaser and Strauss.[7] However, many authors still refer to grounded theory as the constant comparative method.

?

What is a theory, and how will I know one when I see it?

Good question! A theory is a set of statements, hypotheses, or propositions that explain a particular phenomenon or process.[8] Theories come in many forms. Those that are more formal are associated with a label or a researcher's name. For example, Bandura's social learning theory is often referred to as Social Learning Theory. Less formal theories are displayed as simple statements or hypotheses.

Focus

Grounded theory seeks to explain what is occurring in a social context and aims to develop a theory.[9] Therefore, it focuses on social processes. The example of the study by Pitney and Ehlers[10] focuses on process by examining the way in which athletic training students are mentored. Moreover, the study examined in Chapter 2 focuses on how athletic trainers were socialized into their roles in high schools.

Focusing on process generates research questions such as, "How are students mentored to conduct research during undergraduate kinesiology programs?" or "How do exercise physiologists formulate their perceptions of obesity?" A rigorous form of inquiry must be used to generate a theory.

Methods

Grounded theory uses many forms of data, but participant interviews are most common. Alternative, but very viable, methods are the use of documents and observations as primary data sources.[11]

The steps for data analysis are very prescriptive, and the stages of analysis are clearly identifiable.[12,13] In grounded theory, the researchers concentrate first on coding the available data as they are collected. Coding is the process of identifying and labeling pieces of information, concepts, or experiences that pertain to the research questions. The first stage of this procedure is called *open coding*.[13] Open coding involves creating and organizing categories, and is similar to the thematizing process identified in Chapter 4.

The categories that emerge from the data during open coding are "an essential aspect of transforming raw data into theoretical constructions of social processes."[4] The process of open coding also identifies subcategories. Constant comparison is an important aspect of this process.[6] As the name suggests, researchers continuously compare data codes for similar information in order to create distinct categories.

Strauss and Corbin[13] identified axial coding as the second stage of analysis. Axial coding is the process of making connections between the categories and subcategories. Researchers must examine several components related to causes, contexts, contingencies, consequences, covariances, and conditions.[12] Researchers ask the following questions to discover these emerging relationships:

- Do the instances in one category seem to cause or create instances from another category?
- Does the context of the study influence the events or processes that have been discovered? If so, how?
- Are there consequences when an event occurs? If so, what are they?
- Are there contingences that occur only when another event unfolds?
- When one situation changes, does another change occur?
- Under what conditions do experiences and processes occur?

By asking these questions, researchers identify the relationships between the emergent categories. This process of coding helps researchers conceptualize and explain what is happening with the study's participants.

The selective coding process is the last phase of analysis. In selective coding, researchers identify a core category to which all other categories are related. They develop a set of explanatory concepts when they describe the relationship between other categories and the central category. Thus, the theory emerges.[14] The creation of theory requires a great deal of thought, logic, and creativity from the researchers as they fully examine relationships in the data.

Products

The name *grounded theory* foreshadows its product—a theory, or set of explanatory concepts, is produced. The product of grounded theory is an understanding of what is happening with an issue under investigation.

The theory must be based, or grounded, in data obtained during the investigation. Although information from previous studies may inform the process, researchers must rely on data from interviews and observations to develop a theoretical explanation of the process they studied.

Many researchers choose to portray their theories as a model. Models or diagrams can give a visual picture of what has occurred and how events relate to one another.

May I complete a grounded-theory study without developing a theory at the end?

No! If you follow a specific method, you should hold true to its tenets. You have not finished a grounded-theory study until you have formulated a theory based on the data you collected.

Purpose Statement

Grounded theory studies typically look to understand processes that occur. Here is an example of a purpose statement that would direct you toward a grounded-theory study: "The purpose of this … investigation is to understand the process by which clinical decision making is learned by athletic training students."[14] As a more recent example, Sbaraini, Carter, Evans, and Blinkhorn[15] had the following purpose: "We used grounded theory methodology to investigate social processes in private dental practices in New South Wales (NSW), Australia." A subsequent research question might be: "In what way do interactions with coaches influence the clinical decision making of athletic training students?"[14]

ETHNOGRAPHY

Because ethnography is rooted in anthropology, it may conjure up images of exploring the cultures of remote people in a secluded land. From a more contemporary perspective, researchers may find cultures and subcultures everywhere: in hospitals, outpatient rehabilitation clinics, physical education classes, or athletic-training education programs.

Focus

Ethnographic qualitative research involves describing and interpreting a group's culture.[16] Cultural aspects of interest to ethnographers include a group's beliefs, values, and knowledge. Culture tends to be "coded in symbols, the meaning of which have to be learned, be it language or [behavior]."[17]

To clarify the focus further, ethnographic studies attempt to understand how groups create and negotiate meaning, how relationships develop between people, or even how people create and institute policy[18] Additionally, ethnographers hope to identify the structure of a culture, such as whether a hierarchy exists, what the punishments and rewards are like, and whether there are any rituals. Ahlstedt, Lindvall, Holmstrom, and Athlin[19] conducted an ethnographic study exploring the work culture and why registered nurses continue to work, despite being in very stressful environments. The authors observed the workdays of nurses over a long time and identified interpersonal support that nourished and motivated the nurses in the work setting, motivation to solve complex problems and make progress in the clinical setting, and being able to work independently as key motivational aspects of the workplace that influenced nurses to stay in their roles.

To learn aspects of a culture, researchers must become part of the group they are studying.[17] You cannot learn a culture from the outside looking in; you must examine it from the inside looking around. Culture shapes who we are and how we think. Therefore, when researchers conduct an ethnography, they attempt to truly gain an insider's perspective by learning norms and attempting to understand the "... social world of people."[17]

Methods

Many ethnographers will use all types of data, including quantitative data. For example, a researcher immersed in a work setting, such as a hospital, may fully describe the size of the facility, the demographic profile of workers, and even the number of various personnel, along with the demographics of the community in which the hospital is situated. Combining census data with qualitative data allowed the authors to provide a rich description of the setting.

Fieldwork is the cornerstone of the ethnographic research method and includes going to the cultural setting to collect data. Ethnographers visit settings and stay for prolonged periods to observe and interview. Due to the extensive period of enculturation, researchers may have difficulty gaining access to the environment. The ethnographer therefore must be adept at negotiation.

Most ethnographers place more emphasis on observation as a method for collecting qualitative data. Although it is important to learn about participants' beliefs and values by interviewing them, ethnographers want to observe these qualities in a natural setting. The forms of observations discussed in Chapter 4 are relevant to ethnographic studies. Spradley,[20] a leading ethnographer, suggests that researchers begin observation by simply describing the physical setting and participants. Descriptive observations will soon lead to focused observations in which researchers deliberately identify what they need in order to answer the research question. Finally, the observation becomes more selective in nature as the researchers identify activities, events, and specific locations for future observations that will address the study's purpose. Think of this process as gaining a sense of the whole before looking at a culture's parts.

Researchers should conduct an open, broad observation before focusing attention on specific aspects to attain the openness of observation associated with ethnography.[21] In other words, researchers should not bring preconceived notions to the task of collecting data. Instead, they must be open to true discovery about how people interact with others in the group.[21]

Another key aspect of the ethnographic method is the use of field notes. Field notes involve logging or documenting what is observed and learned about the cultural setting. Ethnographers also note what their observations mean in the broader cultural context. Bogden and Biklen[22] describe field notes as "the written account of what the researcher hears, sees, experiences, and thinks in the course of collecting and reflecting on the data in a qualitative study."

The structure of field notes varies from researcher to researcher, but all must record the following 2 components:

1. A description of what has occurred
2. What this event means for the broader research purpose

Of all the many forms of qualitative research, ethnography is perhaps the least structured. The quality of being both systematic and flexible is exemplified by ethnography because researchers explore a culture that they do not know. Ethnography has been described as "… an unstructured approach to research where the researcher needs to be explorative and flexible to 'follow the data,' making decisions throughout the research process about what, where, and when data will be collected."[17] As personal relationships are discovered and social interactions unfold, the researchers may need more time to understand important facets of the findings.

? *I understand that long-term fieldwork is important, but is it possible to wear out my welcome at the research site?*

You must remain culturally entrenched until you have gained the insight necessary to thoroughly explain and describe the culture. In this case, time is measured in understanding rather than in hours.

Products

Every form of research has an outcome. In ethnography, the outcome presented in an article is a rich description of a specific culture and the social dynamics that occur. The written presentation of an ethnography is largely in narrative form. As a reader, you should expect rich explanations of the culture or subculture that include information related to the physical environment, interpersonal relationships, hierarchy, rituals, norms, and values of a group.

Purpose Statement

Here is a brief example of a purpose statement, drawing from Ahlstedt and colleagues[19] that would lead a researcher toward an ethnographic study:

Therefore, the aim of the study was to explore registered nurses' workday events in relation to inner work life theory to better understand what influences registered nurses to remain in work.

PHENOMENOLOGY

Phenomenology is both a research method and philosophy. The philosophical base draws from the pioneering works of Merleau-Ponty, Husserl, and Heidegger.[23] The philosophical tenets are well beyond the scope of this text, but the final section of this chapter recommends additional sources.

Focus

The focus of phenomenology is how people experience and draw meaning from their worlds. As the term implies, researchers are interested in how participants experience a specific phenomenon. A phenomenological research study focuses on the meaning that several participants assign to a particular experience.[24] Therefore, phenomenology focuses on describing the essence of experience.

The term *essence* means that researchers search for the fundamental nature, real meaning, or core aspects of the phenomenon. The process distills a set of experiences until all that is left is what really matters most, which helps describe a participant's life, world, and perception of a phenomenon.

Phenomena are plentiful in our daily lives. Learning, loving, caring, and hoping are all examples. In athletic training, researchers could frame *loss of function* and *disability* as phenomena and explore the experiences of living with a disability from the perspective of an injured athlete.

Methods

The methods of phenomenology have been described by well-respected researchers, including Giorgi[25] and Colaizzi.[26] Giorgi explained the phenomenological method as having 4 steps, whereas Colaizzi identified 7 steps. Lemon and Taylor[27] explained the phenomenological method. We have combined these authors' work to capture the method with the following steps:

1. Bracketing
2. Collecting data
3. Analyzing data
4. Transforming data
5. Sharing the story

Bracketing

Bracketing means that researchers first attempt to set aside their own beliefs, thoughts, and preconceived notions about the phenomenon under investigation.[28] Researchers bracket so that they can learn about the participants' perceptions without including their own ideas in the study. Lemon and Taylor[27] describe this process as suspending your previous knowledge of a phenomenon by engaging in deep self-reflection. As Lancy[16] suggests, researchers should avoid making assumptions in this type of study. They must enter the process with an open mind to learn the true complexities of a phenomenon.

We suggest writing down your thoughts about the phenomenon. The writing process is closely linked to the thought process, so it is a great way to bracket your perceptions. At the very least, if you identify your biases ahead of time, you will recognize them if they enter the process of data analysis. Take time to search your beliefs and write why the topic is important to you, what you think you know about it, and what experiences you have with it.

Collecting Data

Interviewing is the most critical and noteworthy method of data collection in phenomenology.[29] Researchers collect data from individuals who have experienced the phenomenon, so they must use very purposeful interview criteria. Once they have identified participants, they conduct an interview or series of interviews.

When interviewing participants, you must cover 2 broad aspects that are based on the works of Moustakas[30] and summarized by Creswell[24]:

1. How has the participant experienced the phenomenon?
2. What has influenced their perception of and experience with the phenomenon?

Seidman[31] advocated conducting three 90-minute interviews with participants. Each interview focuses on a different aspect of the experience:

1. Focused life history
2. Details of the experience
3. Reflection on the meaning

I am using Seidman's approach to interviewing, but I am not able to conduct a third interview with one of the participants. How should I proceed?

Use any data you have already collected that contributes to an understanding of the past and present aspects of the phenomenon. Be sure to document your change in procedures.

Analyzing and Transforming Data

The analyzing and transforming steps of the phenomenological process are different, but difficult to separate. The analysis step typically follows a process similar to the one described in Chapter 3. In phenomenology, researchers identify any statements made by the participants that provide information about the phenomenon. Phenomenologists next thematize these statements, which are often called *meaning units*. The goal of organizing the meaning units and creating themes is to manage information that will ultimately enable the researcher to describe the phenomenon.

The transforming step attempts to distill the phenomenon down to its essence, or the meaning of the experience. Researchers first describe the participants' experiences based on the emergent themes. Next, they explain how the participants experienced the phenomenon and what it means to them. To transform the data, researchers capture the expressions and language that participants use to describe their experiences. In this process, researchers must ask, "How can I describe what I have learned in a manner that captures its essence and does justice to the participant's experience, yet presents the general meaning of the phenomenon?"[23]

Sharing the Story

When entering this final step of the process, researchers must answer this key question: "From the perspective of the participants, how can this phenomenon be described to others?" Researchers must bring the experience to life for the readers with supporting quotes to illustrate the essence of the phenomenon. At this point, researchers must take the results and descriptions back to the participants for review and approval. This practice is very similar to the process of member checking.[26]

Products

This form of qualitative research generates a rich and exhaustive description of a given experience and uncovers unknown aspects of the phenomenon. For example, Goodwin and Compton[32] unveiled a series of paradoxes that occurred in the lives of women with disabilities, including "the belief that a high quality of life is dependent upon physical wellness and independence and what these young women anticipate for their futures as they age." If your interests lead you toward a phenomenological investigation, we suggest you take the advice of Lancy[16] and select a complex phenomenon about which little is known and critical questions still exist. An example of a complex topic is the experience of pain, which Dudgeon, Gerrard, Jensen, Rhodes, and Tyler[33] investigated in their study titled "Physical Disability and the Experience of Chronic Pain." Using a phenomenological method for less complex topics may "capture too much; it is wasteful.[16] In other words, both the researcher and the research would be better served with a different theoretical approach. Therefore, articulate the phenomenon of interest to your colleagues or advisors, who can help you ascertain whether the topic is complex enough to warrant such an intense investigation.

? **Do I have to select one approach to qualitative research?**

No. Although some researchers have stated that using a specific form of inquiry leads to a higher level of sophistication and may "… convey a level of methodological expertise,"[24] we respectfully disagree. You can have a substantial level of rigor and obtain a great deal of insight and understanding with a basic or generic interpretive study. Your expertise and the study's sophistication will be apparent in how you plan and execute the study.

Purpose Statement

Here is a brief example of a research purpose statement from Kinsella, Park, Appiagyei, Change, and Chow[34] who studied the experience of ethical tension in occupational therapy practice from the perspectives of students: "The purpose of this study was to examine the nature of ethical tensions witnessed or experienced by occupational therapy students during practice education."

ADDITIONAL TYPES OF QUALITATIVE RESEARCH

This last section focuses on 3 additional forms of qualitative research. Although they are less common in literature on physical activity and the health professions, you may encounter a qualitative case study, action research study, or narrative inquiry. You should have a basic understanding of each type.

Qualitative Case Studies

Qualitative case studies are intense investigations of a single unit of study, or a *bounded system*. Examples include one person, one educational program, one school, a single class, a nursing ward, a hospital, or a wellness center.

Merriam[1] states that researchers may select a bounded system because it is the focus of an identified issue or concern. The bounded system may also be unique in some way. Qualitative case studies use many forms of data to understand what is happening, including observations, documents, and interviews. The product is a rich description of the case and an explanation of how it operates.

Please note that we use the term *qualitative case study* very purposefully. Some case studies, especially in medicine, rely on quantitative data, like diagnostic tests, to paint a clear picture of what a patient has experienced and how the treatment was effective. Case studies use many forms of data, not just qualitative information. Therefore, you must be very clear about the design you have chosen.

A positive aspect of conducting a case study is that you will not need to work with any participants beyond those involved with the bounded system. In other words, you only need to collect data as it relates to your case. If you decide to conduct a qualitative case study of a unique adapted physical education program for students with multiple sclerosis, you would interview the students, parents, instructors, and administrators. Your observations would be limited to that single program. You would not need to observe other programs or conduct interviews with anyone who is not involved with the case.

A limitation of qualitative case studies is that their findings are rarely transferable. However, you shouldn't feel too apologetic about this limitation. Qualitative case studies tend to focus on unique programs, special concerns, and interesting situations. How they compare to other contexts may be irrelevant; your goal is to vividly describe this case so others can learn about it. Readers can make their own decisions about how to use the findings.

Action Research

Action research is a very practical form of inquiry that is designed to produce a specific outcome, change, or improvement in the very setting in which it is conducted.[35] It is systematically conducted by practitioners, such as clinicians or teachers, to gather information about how procedures are performed (ie, how teachers teach or how patients are treated) and how context influences outcomes.[35,36] Stringer[35] elucidated the following characteristics of action research:

- *Change*: Practitioners work on changing their behaviors to improve their practice.
- *Reflection*: Practitioners reflect on, think about, and theorize about their roles and functions.
- *Participation*: Participants change their own practices and behaviors, not those of others.
- *Sharing*: Participants share their perspectives on the context with others.
- *Understanding*: The study enhances understanding of different perspectives.
- *Practice*: Participants apply their findings to their practice.

Action research most commonly employs qualitative data collection and analysis because of the depth of understanding that can be obtained about a specific context. Remember that the focus of action research is changing and improving practice.

Narrative Inquiry

Researchers use narrative inquiry to gain a deep and rich understanding of participants' experiences. The main method is listening to participants' life stories. Narrative researchers believe hearing the stories of others helps you best understand the meaning that participants assign to their experiences.

Because narrative inquiry focuses on life experiences, some researchers tend to link it with life histories, biographies, and even autobiographies.[2] Shank[37] states that narrative inquiry uses strategies of data analysis that are similar to the grounded theory method and sometimes employ formal linguistic analysis. However, as Schram[2] suggests, narrative inquiry is often viewed as running counter to other methods of analysis that break qualitative data down into codes and then regroup it to form interpretations. When conducting narrative analysis, remember to share your participants' stories in a way that represents what has occurred in their lives. Consider the holistic nature of their stories by presenting lengthy block quotes that capture the meaning of their experiences.

SUMMARY

Many forms of qualitative research exist. The majority of this text addresses the general approach to qualitative research. Researchers who choose a specific type of qualitative research must attend to its foci, methods, and products. Grounded theory examines social processes and seeks to generate a theory or theories. Ethnography focuses on understanding a particular culture. Phenomenology focuses on how participants have experienced a specific phenomenon. Although these 3 forms of qualitative research are common, many additional forms exist. Some researchers mix these forms to achieve a unique research purpose.

CONTINUE YOUR EDUCATIONAL JOURNEY

LEARN THROUGH ACTIVITY

1. Create a table that lists the forms of qualitative research in a vertical column on the left and the research focus, method, and outcomes in a horizontal row across the top. Fill in the answers for the intersecting cells to create a useful summary.

2. Search for and read a grounded theory, ethnography, and phenomenological study in your health care discipline. Examine each article and identify the research purpose and questions used to guide the methods. How could the purpose of each study be changed to warrant using another form of inquiry?

CHECK YOUR KNOWLEDGE

1. This form of qualitative research focuses on understanding an existing culture:
   a. Ethnography
   b. Grounded theory
   c. Phenomenology
   d. a and c
   e. a and b

2. This form of qualitative research produces an exhaustive description of participants' lived experiences:
   a. Ethnography
   b. Grounded theory
   c. Phenomenology
   d. a and c
   e. a and b

3. This form of qualitative research relies on long-term field observation to gain insight and understanding:
   a. Ethnography
   b. Grounded theory
   c. Phenomenology
   d. a and c
   e. a and b

4. This form of qualitative research uses rigorous and systematic procedures of coding to create a set of explanatory concepts:
   a. Ethnography
   b. Grounded theory
   c. Phenomenology
   d. a and c
   e. a and b

5. This form of qualitative research often produces a conceptual model:
   a. Ethnography
   b. Grounded theory
   c. Phenomenology
   d. a and c
   e. a and b

6. Categories are developed in which step of grounded theory?
   a. Open coding
   b. Axial coding
   c. Selective coding
   d. a and c
   e. a and b

7. Which of the following forms of research emphasizes a bounded system?

   a. Narrative inquiry

   b. Phenomenology

   c. Action research

   d. Qualitative case study

   e. None of the above

8. A health teacher wants to change a unit on drug and alcohol abuse to raise awareness about the dangers these substances pose for society. What form of inquiry would best serve this purpose?

   a. Narrative inquiry

   b. Phenomenology

   c. Action research

   d. Qualitative case study

   e. None of the above

THINK ABOUT IT

1. You are planning to study the conflict between the work and home lives of athletic trainers. What form of qualitative research might best achieve this purpose? Why?

2. You are conducting an ethnography to understand how highly competitive sporting environments influence how medical decisions are made. How would you gain access to this environment? How would you collect and analyze data? Whom would you wish to observe and interview? What other forms of data would you wish to collect and analyze?

MAKE A STRETCH

We recommend reviewing these examples of various forms of qualitative research from various health professions:

Grounded Theory

- Jette D, Bertoni A, Coots R, et al. Clinical instructors' perceptions of behaviors that comprise entry-level clinical performance in physical therapist students: a qualitative study. *Phys Ther.* 2007;87(7):833-843.
- Licqurish S, Seibold C. Applying a contemporary grounded theory methodology. *Nurse Res.* 2011;18:4,11-16.

Phenomenology

- Kinsella EA, Park AJ, Appiagyei J, Chang E, Chow D. Through the eyes of students: ethical tensions in occupational therapy practice. *Can J Occup Ther.* 2008;75(3):176-183.
- Schmid T. Meanings of creativity within occupational therapy practice. *Aust Occup Ther J.* 2004;51:80-88.

Ethnography

- Ahlstedt C, Lindvall CE, Holmstrom IK, Athlin AM. What makes registered nurses remain in work? An ethnographic study. *Int J Nurs Stud.* 2019;89:32-38.
- Hunter CL, Spence K, McKenna K, Iedema R. Learning how we learn: an ethnographic study in a neonatal intensive care unit. *J Adv Nurs.* 2008;62(6):657-664.

Case Study

- McGarvey HE, Chambers MG, Boore JRP. The influence of context on role behaviors of perioperative nurses. *AORN J.* 2004;80(6):1103-1119.

Action Research

- Khunti K, Stone MA, Bankart J et al. Primary prevention of type-2 diabetes and heart disease: action research in secondary schools serving an ethnically diverse UK population. *J Public Health.* 2007;30(1),:30-37.

Narrative Analysis

- Evans J, Penney D. Levels on the playing field: the social construction of physical "ability" in the physical education curriculum. *Phys Ed Sport Peda.* 2008;13(1):31-47.

REFERENCES

1. Merriam SB. *Qualitative Research and Case Study Applications in Education.* 2nd ed. San Francisco, CA: Jossey-Bass; 1998.
2. Schram TH. *Conceptualizing and Proposing Qualitative Research.* 2nd ed. Upper Saddle River, NJ: Pearson Merrill Prentice Hall; 2006.
3. Holloway I, ed. *Qualitative Research in Health Care.* Berkshire, England: Open University Press; 2005.
4. Kendall J. Axial coding and the grounded theory controversy. *Western J Nurs Res.* 1999;21:743-757.
5. Bluff R. Grounded theory: the methodology. In Holloway I, ed. *Qualitative Research in Health Care.* Berkshire, England: Open University Press; 2005:147-165.
6. Glaser BG, Strauss AL. *The Discovery of Grounded Theory.* Hawthorne, NY: Aldine; 1967.
7. Hallberg LRM. The "core category" of grounded theory: making constant comparisons. *Int J Qual Stud Health Well-being.* 2006;1:141-148.
8. Ary D, Cheser Jacobs LC, Razavieh A. *Introduction to Research in Education.* 6th ed. Belmont, CA: Wadsworth; 2002.
9. Annells M. Grounded theory method: philosophical perspectives, paradigm of inquiry, and postmodernism. *Qualitative Health Res.* 1996;6:379-394.
10. Pitney WA, Ehlers GG. A grounded theory study of the mentoring process involved with undergraduate athletic training students. *J Athl Train.* 2004;39(4):344-351.

11. Pandit NR. The creation of theory: a recent application of the grounded theory method. *Qual Rep.* 1996;2(4):1-15.

12. Glaser B. *Theoretical Sensitivity: Advances in the Methodology of Grounded Theory.* Mill Valley, CA: Sociology Press; 1978.

13. Strauss AL, Corbin JM. *Basics of Qualitative Research: Grounded Theory Procedures and Techniques.* Newbury Park, CA: Sage; 1990.

14. Pitney WA, Parker J. Qualitative research applications in athletic training. *J Athl Train.* 2002;37(4 suppl):S168-S173.

15. Sbaraini A, Carter SM, Evans RW, Blinkhorn A. How to do a grounded theory study: a worked example of a study of dental practices. *BMC Med Res Methodol.* 2011;11:128.

16. Lancy DF. *Qualitative Research in Education: An Introduction to the Major Traditions.* White Plains, NY: Longman; 1993.

17. Sharkey S, Larsen JA. Ethnographic exploration: participation and meaning in everyday life. In Holloway I, ed. *Qualitative Research in Health Care.* Berkshire, England: Open University Press; 2005:168-190.

18. Beach D. From fieldwork to theory and representation in ethnography. In Troman G, Jeffrey B, Walford G, eds. *Methodological Issues and Practices in Ethnography.* Boston, MA: Elsevier; 2005:1-17.

19. Ahlstedt C, Lindvall CE, Holmstrom IK, Athlin AM. What makes registered nurses remain in work? An ethnographic study. *Int J Nurs Stud.* 2019;89:32-38.

20. Spradley JP. *Participant Observation.* New York, NY: Holt, Rinehart and Winston; 1980.

21. Baszanger I, Dodier N. Ethnography: relating the part to the whole. In Silverman D, ed. *Qualitative Research: Theory, Method and Practice.* Thousand Oaks, CA: Sage; 1997:9-34.

22. Bogdan RC, Biklen SK. *Qualitative Research for Education: An Introduction to Theories and Methods.* 5th ed. Boston, MA: Allyn & Bacon; 2007.

23. Todres L. Clarifying the life-world: descriptive phenomenology. In Holloway I, ed. *Qualitative Research in Health Care.* Berkshire, England: Open University Press; 2005:104-124.

24. Creswell JW. *Qualitative Inquiry & Research Design: Choosing Among Five Approaches.* 2nd ed. Thousand Oaks, CA: Sage; 2007.

25. Giorgi A. *Phenomenology and Psychological Research.* Pittsburgh, PA: Duquesne University Press; 1985.

26. Colaizzi PF. Psychological research as the phenomenologist views it. In Valle RS, King M, eds. *Existential-Phenomenological Alternatives for Psychology.* New York, NY: Oxford University Press; 1978:48-71.

27. Lemon N, Taylor H. Caring in casualty: the phenomenology of nursing care. In Hayes N, ed. *Doing Qualitative Analysis in Psychology.* Hove, England: Psychology Press; 1997:227-244.

28. Byrne MM. Understanding life experiences through a phenomenological approach to research. *AORN J.* 2001;73:830-832.

29. Wimpeny P, Gass J. Interviewing in phenomenology and grounded theory: is there a difference? *J Adv Nurs.* 2000;31(6):1485-1492.

30. Moustakas C. *Phenomenological Research Methods.* Thousand Oaks, CA: Sage; 1994.

31. Seidman IE. *Interviewing as Qualitative Research: A Guide for Researchers in Education and the Social Sciences.* New York, NY: Teachers College Press; 1991.

32. Goodwin DL, Compton SG. Physical activity experiences of women aging with disabilities. *Adapted Phys Activity Quart.* 2004;21:122-138.

33. Dudgeon B, Gerrard BC, Jensen MP, Rhodes LA, Tyler EJ. Physical disability and the experience of chronic pain. *Archives Phys Med Rehab.* 2002;83:229-235.

34. Kinsella EA, Park AJ, Appiagyei J, Chang E, Chow D. Through the eyes of students: ethical tensions in occupational therapy practice. *Canadian J Occupational Ther.* 2008;75(3):176-183.

35. Stringer E. *Action Research in Education.* Upper Saddle River, NJ: Pearson Merrill Prentice Hall; 2004.

36. Mills GE. *Action Research: A Guide for the Teacher Researcher.* 3rd ed. Upper Saddle River, NJ: Pearson Merrill Prentice Hall; 2007.

37. Shank GD. *Qualitative Research: A Personal Skills Approach.* 2nd ed. Upper Saddle River, NJ: Pearson Merrill Prentice Hall; 2006.

Mixed Methods Research Design

Christianne M. Eason, PhD, ATC

LEARNING OBJECTIVES

Readers will be able to do the following:
1. Define mixed methods research.
2. Describe rationales supporting the use of mixed methods research.
3. Differentiate between the 6 common mixed methods research designs.
4. Articulate the importance of mixed methods research designs in the health professions research.

DEFINING MIXED METHODS RESEARCH

As highlighted in a 2015 editorial,[1] almost every interaction between a clinician and a patient involves the collection and incorporation of number (quantitative) and word (qualitative) information. A typical interaction between a health care practitioner in any setting and their patient will start with the clinician asking how the patient is feeling. The patient will respond with words that reflect his or her perceptions of how he or she is feeling, and the next step will be for the clinician to take vital signs or to review laboratory tests or reports, which generally consist of numbers that indicate any deviation from normal values. As pointed out by Fawcett,[1] these typical interactions are actually sophisticated ways to collect data and represent single-case mixed methods research. Mixed methods research is defined as "the collection or analysis of both quantitative and qualitative data in a single study in which the data are collected concurrently or sequentially, are given a priority, and involve integration of the data at one or more stages in the process

Pitney WA, Parker J, Mazerolle Singe S, Potteiger K.
Qualitative Research in the Health Professions (pp 109-123).
© 2020 Taylor & Francis Group.

of research."[2] Mixed methods research should be considered a third research paradigm in addition to quantitative and qualitative methods.

In mixed methods research design, the qualitative component is referred to as *QUAL* or *qual*, and this signifies the data are words. The quantitative component is referred to as *QUAN* or *quan*, and this signifies the data are numbers. The uppercase is used when the study is primarily QUAL or QUAN, whereas lowercase qual and quan are used to indicate which portion of the study was supplementary. This lettering system for representing different mixed methods procedures was developed by Morse.[3,4] In mixed methods research designs, qualitative and quantitative methods and data are combined so weaknesses in one can be offset by strengths in the other. Some methods, which will be discussed later, are designed so that either qualitative or quantitative data are prioritized, whereas other study designs choose to prioritize both. Mixed methods research designs are used by researchers in various disciplines and have become increasingly popular among social science and allied health scholars. It should be considered a stand-alone research design and is ideal for collaborative practice among researchers.

HISTORICAL ORIGINS OF MIXED METHODS RESEARCH

The use of multiple data collection methods has been used in some of the earliest social science and allied health care research. One of the earliest examples of mixed methods research was a validation study of psychological traits published in 1959.[5] The authors focused on collecting multiple quantitative data; however, they encouraged the use of multiple methods and the collection of multiple forms of data in their work. Essentially, they were advocating for *triangulation*, which is a term borrowed from military naval science that illustrates the use of multiple reference points in order to locate the exact position of some object. Their advocacy of data triangulation was suggestive that quantitative and qualitative data could be complementary.

In 1979, Reichardt and Cook[6] argued that different research methods were compatible. They contended that philosophical paradigms and research methods are not inherently linked by citing several examples that highlighted that quantitative procedures are not always objective and qualitative procedures are not always subjective. There are those who oppose the use of mixed methods research design, arguing that postpositivist worldviews should be combined only with quantitative designs and that naturalistic worldviews should be combined only with qualitative methods. Reichardt and Rallis[7] referred to this as the *paradigm debate*, in which mixed methods research design is viewed as incompatible because certain paradigms and methods just do not fit together. Those who disagree with this viewpoint contend that the generalizability of quantitative findings and the contextual nature of qualitative findings can be taken advantage of in a single research study.[8] Adding further support for the use of mixed methods research design is the pragmatism perspective, which was first associated with mixed methods research design in 1985.[9] Pragmatists believe that you can use diverse approaches and value objective and subjective knowledge[10] and that regardless of circumstances, both methods can be used in a single study.[9]

Numerous rationales support the use of mixed methods research designs. It has been argued by researchers that mixed methods investigations may use converging numeric trends from quantitative data and specific details from qualitative data to better understand specific research problems, obtain quantitative data from a population sample and use those to identify individuals who may expand on results through qualitative data; results from one method may be combined to elaborate on results from the other method in a complementary manner and for the development of new instruments of data collection.[11-14] Regardless of the philosophical perspective, it is important for every researcher to remember that the research question should be the primary factor that underlies the research method.

DESIGNING A MIXED METHODS STUDY

Designing a mixed methods study follows many similar steps to those taken in any traditional research method. The steps must include establishing a purpose of the study, forming research questions, and deciding on the type of data to collect. The most apparent reason for using a mixed methods research design is because the research question or research problem necessitates it. It is important to keep in mind that there are some weaknesses of mixed methods research designs. These include (1) the time required to complete data collection and analysis, (2) needing to resolve discrepancies that may arise between different types of data, (3) the difficult decision in deciding when to proceed if utilizing a sequential design, and (4) little guidance on transformative methods. Methodologist John Creswell[2,15,16] has suggested that researchers make 4 decisions before moving forward with a mixed methods research design. These decisions should include (1) determining the implementation of data collection, (2) deciding which method will take priority during data collection and analysis, (3) how data will be integrated, and (4) determining if a theoretical perspective will be used.

Determining how data will be prioritized and implemented is a very important decision when planning a mixed methods research design. Priority refers to the relative emphasis given to the 2 types of data: unequal or equal.[17] Unequal priority occurs if a researcher emphasizes one form more than the other, starts with one form as the major component of the study, or collects one form of data in more detail than the other.[18] Implementation refers to the order in which the data are collected: sequentially or concurrently.[17] Tables 8-1 and 8-2 highlight the many potential choices in this step, which were originally illustrated in a 2005 article on mixed methods research design in counseling psychology.[19] Researchers also need to determine how they will analyze the data. The analysis of data collected via mixed methods research designs is an iterative process with the goal of combining or cross-validating the qualitative and quantitative data. Specific to mixed methods research design, data analysis can be classified as parallel, conversion, sequential, or integrated.[20]

? *I am planning a research study and believe mixed methods is the best approach based on my research question. Which of the forms of data, qualitative or quantitative, should I put first in the study and emphasize in my data analysis?*

The answer and your decision regarding data priority will depend on the goal of the study. If the goal is to explain results, a researcher should collect quantitative data first and then qualitative data.

TABLE 8-1		
UNEQUAL EMPHASES IN CONCURRENT AND SEQUENTIAL MIXED METHODS DESIGN		
	QUALITATIVE EMPHASIS	**QUANTITATIVE EMPHASIS**
CONCURRENT	QUAL + quan	QUAN + qual
	quan + QUAL	Qual + QUAN
SEQUENTIAL	QUAL → quan	QUAN → qual
	quan → QUAL	qual → QUAN
Adapted from Hanson WE, Creswell JW, Plano Clark VL, Petski KS, Creswell JD. Mixed methods research designs in counseling psychology. *J Couns Psychol.* 2005;52(2):22-235.		

TABLE 8-2	
EQUAL EMPHASES IN CONCURRENT AND SEQUENTIAL MIXED METHODS DESIGN	
CONCURRENT	QUAN + QUAL or QUAL + QUAN
SEQUENTIAL	QUAN → QUAL or QUAL → QUAN
Adapted from Hanson WE, Creswell JW, Plano Clark VL, Petski KS, Creswell JD. Mixed methods research designs in counseling psychology. *J Couns Psychol.* 2005;52(2):22-235.	

Mixed Methods Research Data Analysis

In the parallel approach, which is the most widely used,[16,20] qualitative and quantitative data analysis are 2 separate processes. Conclusions regarding each separate type of data are drawn independently and then both forms of data are considered together. The goal of parallel analysis is often data triangulation. Conversion analysis is a process in which qualitative data are quantified by transforming them into codes or counts. If qualitative data are quantified via numeric coding, then these data can be merged with the original quantitative data. Quantitative data could also be turned into words, which is known as *qualitizing*, by creating themes based on numerical survey data. In a sequential analysis each of the data types are dependent on the other in a way that the results of one data set are used to plan the next data set. Using this type of analysis is very fluid, as the phases of analysis evolve as the study develops. Typically, with a sequential analysis, the findings of each form of data are presented in the results and the interpretation of how the qualitative data inform the quantitative data (or vice versa) occurs in the discussion section. Integrated data analysis can include a combination of the other 3 analysis procedures and is typically used in the more advanced mixed methods research classifications (eg, embedded, transformative, multiphase) that are described in the next section. Integrative analysis is the interactive mixing of quantitative and qualitative data and is characterized as being iterative and reciprocal. Whichever approach is selected, it is essential that interpretations of the data include the convergence or divergence of mixed methods research design data.

It is also important to remember that convergence is not the ultimate goal of analyses and mixed methods research designs. Divergent conclusions between data sources are a major advantage of mixed methods research designs, as they can provide great value.

Mixed Methods Research Design Classifications

Several classification systems have been developed to identify the various typologies of mixed methods research designs. Initially, in the first edition of their textbook, Creswell and Plano Clark[21] proposed 4 designs for mixed methods research: (1) exploratory, (2) explanatory, (3) triangulation, and (4) embedded designs. The main difference between each design was timing and emphasis, referring to the concurrent or sequential data collection and then determining which component would be emphasized. In the second edition of their textbook[16] they refined the classification system to define 6 primary types of designs,[22] which include sequential exploratory, sequential explanatory, convergent parallel, transformative, multiphase, and embedded. Each design differs in regard to its use of theoretical lens, implementation approach, and data analysis and integration. Although these differences may seem subtle, it is important to understand the differences among them. The variance in these typologies highlights the technical challenges of implementing the timing of qualitative and quantitative methods and the emphasis placed on each method. An explanation follows of Creswell and Plano Clark's[22] typology of mixed methods design grouped into 3 categories: (1) sequential designs, (2) concurrent designs, and (3) concurrent or sequential.

Sequential Designs

Sequentially designed studies involve collecting one form of data and then collecting the second form of data. This data collection will usually occur over time, and it is important for researchers to determine when each phase of data collection will begin.

As the name implies, a sequential explanatory design is useful if the goal of a study is to explain relationships or results. For example, a research group wants to examine the impact of a recently implemented type 2 diabetes prevention program and their research questions include the following: Is a prevention program effective in reducing cases of type 2 diabetes? What are the perceptions and opinions of community members who are participating in the program? In a sequential explanatory design quantitative data are collected and analyzed, then qualitative data. Usually, priority is unequal and is given to the quantitative data, with the qualitative data used to supplement the quantitative data. In the example regarding a type 2 diabetes prevention program, researchers could first collect quantitative data on blood glucose levels and other biomarkers related to diabetes in addition to collecting data relating to diagnosis rates. After reviewing the quantitative data, researchers could conduct focus groups with participants to gain their perspective and determine why the program was or was not effective. Analysis of the data is typically connected, and integration of the data occurs during interpretation of the data and in the discussion.

A sequential exploratory study design involves qualitative data collected and analyzed first, followed by quantitative data. Additionally, priority is unequal and given to the qualitative data. These types of designs are optimal if the goal of a study is to explore relationships when variables are not known, development of a new test or instrument, or generalizing qualitative findings to a specific population. For example, if a researcher wanted to know the characteristics and attitudes of women athletic trainers who have left the profession and which recruitment strategies would be most effective in recruiting women athletic trainers for a survey research project, as well as how the characteristics and attitudes of women athletic trainers who have left the profession compare to women who remain in the profession, a sequential exploratory study would be ideal. Qualitative data can be collected initially via personal interviews with the intent to uncover the characteristics and attitudes unique to women who have left the athletic training profession to help develop an appropriate questionnaire. A quantitative questionnaire can then be developed based on the qualitative data.

Concurrent Design

Concurrent designs involve collecting both qualitative and quantitative data at the same time. In the convergent parallel design the qualitative and quantitative components are of equal priority and applied independently. The goal of these types of mixed methods study designs are to cross-validate data. If a researcher wants to determine the differences in the dietary behaviors, exercise patterns, and attitudes toward treatment between oncology patients receiving chemotherapy and those receiving radiation treatment, then a convergent parallel design would be optimal. This type of design would allow researchers to collect quantitative data from a questionnaire and collect qualitative data via phone interviews at approximately the same time points. Data collected from both methodologies would then be blended to thoroughly understand the factors under investigation and to determine if there are differences between the patient groups.

Concurrent or Sequential Designs

Concurrent or sequential designs give researchers the flexibility in determining the timing of data collection. Data can be collected at the same time, or one form of data can be collected and then the next. The underlying research purpose and research questions should drive the timing of the data collection.

Embedded research designs, also referred to as *nested research designs*, involve a small amount of either qualitative data or quantitative data to be included within a larger qualitative or quantitative study. These designs can be such that the quantitative methodologies are the priority and a smaller qualitative methodology is implemented at the same time with unequal priority and vice versa. Including open-ended questions to gather qualitative data in a larger quantitative survey is an example of an embedded mixed methods design. Likewise, including a few quantitative questions within a qualitative interview guide would also be an example of an embedded mixed methods design. If researchers are using an existing reliable and valid quantitative survey instrument but may be uncertain if they are truly capturing all of the important attitudes and beliefs that a specific population has, they may decide to incorporate a qualitative open-ended section to collect additional data that will allow participants to describe their perceptions in their own words.

The transformative research design describes any combination of methods conducted in which there is an overarching transformative framework. In these studies it is typically a social problem and the related theories that necessitate the use of both qualitative and quantitative methodologies, with the ultimate goal of solving the underlying social problems. Any of the previously described designs can be applied within the transformative design, so this approach is not a specific design, but rather an ideological or philosophical approach.

A multiphase design is used to describe any combination of methods that are conducted within a complex program of research. This design combines concurrent and sequential data collection over time in order to complete a large study that is multidimensional.

Sampling Procedures

Quantitative research often utilizes probability sampling, which includes subjects being randomly selected from a population with a goal of achieving a representative sample. Recruitment numbers involve selecting a sample large enough to ensure statistical power and to provide the desired representativeness. Qualitative research often uses purposive sampling, which involves selecting a subject based on a specific reason rather than randomly. Sample size numbers do not have a steadfast rule in qualitative research; rather, recruitment is guided by data saturation, the point at which ideas have been exhausted and no new information is being produced. The trade-off is that probability sampling leads to a large breadth of information from a generalizable sample, whereas purposive sampling produces a greater depth of information from a less generalizable sample. Mixed methods research design sampling utilizes a combination of probability and purposive sampling.[20] The main advantage of mixed methods research design sampling is that the weaknesses and shortfalls in one sampling procedure are counterbalanced by strengths in the other. The disadvantage, of course, is the added time and resources required to complete appropriate sampling.

PUTTING IT TOGETHER

Regardless of the type of mixed method design that it is implemented, all mixed methods studies should include a clear purpose statement, research questions, and evident rationale for utilizing both qualitative and quantitative data.[2] The inclusion of a rationale for mixed methods data collection allows a reader to comprehend that the collection of qualitative and quantitative data was intentional and not haphazard. It is recommended that this rationale be stated clearly in the introduction, where it can be specified what the advantages are for using both methods and data and how that will help answer the study's research questions.[19]

Mixed methods study designs require a strong working knowledge of both qualitative and quantitative methods, and because data collection and analysis will often extend over long periods, it is recommended that researchers work in teams.[19] Research teams allow individuals with expertise in one method or the other, or both, to directly design and implement an optimal mixed methods study. This recommendation is echoed in the works of Fawcett, who describes mixed methods research designs as ideal for multidisciplinary research[23] and collaborative practice.[24] The reality is that some researchers and clinicians may have a greater ability to collect, analyze, and interpret qualitative data, whereas others may be more comfortable working with number data.

(?) ***Can mixed methods studies help enhance collaborative practice among researchers?***

Yes. Due to the time required to complete data collection and analysis, in addition to the specialties required to analyze and interpret qualitative and quantitative data, researchers of various research backgrounds can come together to help provide robust answers to research questions.

ILLUSTRATION OF MIXED METHODS RESEARCH DESIGNS

Mixed methods research design studies have been published within the literature of various health professions' in recent years (Table 8-3). Researchers in many disciplines have called for more application of mixed methods research designs within their fields, including, nursing,[1] nutrition and dietetics,[25] counseling psychology,[19,22] speech-language therapy,[26] prehospital research,[27] and physical therapy.[28] In this section, several published studies will be described to illustrate the value of mixed methods research designs within the health professions. In doing so, elements of mixed methods research design, such as implementation, priority, and data analysis, may be easier to understand in context.

Mazerolle, Eason, and Goodman[29] used an embedded design to compare the perspectives of athletic trainers working in 3 different collegiate sports medicine organizational structures regarding work-life balance, role strain, job satisfaction, and retention. Fifty-nine athletic trainers completed the quantitative portion of the study, and 24 athletic trainers participated in the qualitative portion of the study. In this study the authors clearly stated the study's purpose and rationale for using a mixed methods research study design, implemented data collection sequentially (quantitative then qualitative), prioritized the qualitative data, and integrated the data after analyzing them in an interpretation phase. Specifically, quantitative data, in the form of demographic information and Likert scores on 5 different measures, and qualitative data, in the form of tape-recorded one-on-one phone interviews, were analyzed separately and then the results were triangulated. Based on their analyses and triangulation of data, the authors were able to conclude that there were some commonalities among athletic trainers working in all 3 organizational settings, including communication, social support, time management, and effective work-life balance strategies. However, they also noted differences among the models and were able to conclude that athletic trainers working in an athletics model worked more hours, were less satisfied with their pay, believed they had less support from their administrators, and had fewer plans to remain in their current positions. Additional examples of embedded mixed methods research designs can be found in Table 8-3.

Ashton et al[30] used a sequential exploratory design in order to explore the recruitment strategies, content, facilitator characteristics, and delivery mode and program duration and frequency preferences of young males for lifestyle intervention programs. The researchers conducted 10 focus groups involving 61 young men between the ages of 18 and 25. Upon completion of the focus groups, researchers used those results and questions developed from a developmental model to create a cross-sectional online survey. As was previously discussed, qualitative data are prioritized in sequential exploratory designs, and these designs are optimal if the goal is to develop a new test or instrument. The findings of this study confirmed the importance of consulting participants when designing lifestyle intervention programs, and the researchers were able to conclude that future programs for young men should incorporate individualized goals and feedback; resistance training; and information on quick, easy, and cheap meals.

TABLE 8-3

PUBLISHED MIXED METHODS RESEARCH DESIGNS IN MULTIPLE HEALTH PROFESSION DISCIPLINES

FIELD	AUTHORS	PURPOSE STATEMENT	CLASSIFICATION
Athletic training	Mazerolle, Eason, & Goodman (2017)	"To compare athletic trainers' perspectives on work-life balance, role strain, job satisfaction, and retention in collegiate practice settings within various organizational structures."[29(p12)]	Embedded
	Clement, Granquist, & Arvinen-Barrow (2013)	"The current study's primary purpose was to determine (a) perceived psychological responses and coping behaviors athletes may present to athletic trainers, (b) psychosocial strategies athletic trainers currently use with their athletes, (c) psychosocial strategies athletic trainers deem important to learn more about, and (d) athletic trainers' current practices in referring athletes to counseling or sport psychology services."[32(p512)]	Embedded
Nutrition and dietetics	Ashton et al (2017)	"Explore young males' preferences for recruitment strategies, content, format, and facilitator characteristics for future physical activity and nutritional interventions."[30(p1588)]	Sequential exploratory
	Burgermaster et al (2017)	"To determine if classroom context affects childhood obesity prevention programs."[33(p3)]	Multiphase
Nursing	Craft, Christensen, Bakon, & Wirihana (2017)	"To evaluate the implementation, influence, and student perspective of a team-teaching workshop to integrate bioscience theory with clinical nursing practice."[34(p114)]	Sequential explanatory

(continued)

TABLE 8-3 (CONTINUED)

PUBLISHED MIXED METHODS RESEARCH DESIGNS IN MULTIPLE HEALTH PROFESSION DISCIPLINES

FIELD	AUTHORS	PURPOSE STATEMENT	CLASSIFICATION
	Lamont et al (2015)	"To explore intraprofessional collaboration among nursing leadership teams at a tertiary referral hospital in Sydney."[35(p1126)]	Sequential explanatory
	De Meester, Van Bogaert, Clarke, & Bossert (2012)	"To investigate the circumstances of nursing care 8 hours before serious adverse events on medical and surgical nursing units with subsequent in-hospital mortality in order to identify the extent to which these serious adverse events were potentially preventable."[31(p2308)]	Sequential explanatory
Orthopedics	Leggott et al (2016)	"To provide insight into how an innovation in health care is implemented and diffused, the transition from routine use of general anesthesia to peripheral nerve blocks for ambulatory orthopedic surgery was studied."[36(p181)]	Sequential explanatory
Physical therapy	Comer et al (2016)	"To explore factors that might be relevant when designing a triage tool."[37(p900)]	Sequential explanatory
	Hebesberger et al (2016)	"To explore the possibility of robot deployment supporting physical therapy of older adults with advanced dementia."[38(p27-28)]	Convergent parallel
Primary care	Van den Bruel, Jones, Thompson, & Mant (2016)	"To determine the acceptability and impact of C-reactive protein testing in acutely ill children."[39(p382)]	Embedded

De Meester et al[31] conducted a sequential explanatory study on medical and surgical nursing units to investigate the circumstances of nursing care in the hours before a serious adverse event that resulted in an in-hospital mortality. Their goal was to determine the extent to which the serious adverse events were possibly preventable. The researchers completed a retrospective review of 63 patient records of serious adverse events in a teaching hospital where patient death was the final outcome. The data from chart reviews were combined with data regarding the working conditions on the nursing unit at the time of the events. Experts' opinions regarding the preventability of the outcomes were also collected. Results of this study led the researchers to conclude that nurses were often unaware of the deteriorating condition of their patients before the crisis and that the nurse-reported threshold for concern regarding abnormal vital signs suggested they would call for assistance fairly late in a clinical crisis situation. The clinical relevance of this study is apparent, as the results have a direct impact on patient care and highlight the importance of mixed methods research designs in the research.

SUMMARY

Mixed methods research design allows researchers to enrich their results in ways that using only one form of data (qualitative or quantitative) may not allow. The key to the best mixed methods research is the integration, not a simple combination, of qualitative and quantitative data.[15] Ideal health care practice relies on a collection of both word and number information to form the best understanding of the patient's whole health condition.[1] Analogously, utilizing both word and number data in research may help provide researchers with a better understanding of their research questions. In choosing to use a mixed methods research design, it is essential that the researcher is clear in choosing mixed methods and in the selection and description of the study design. Given the parallels between clinical practice and mixed methods research designs, it is recommended that more researchers consider using this tactic.

CONTINUE YOUR EDUCATIONAL JOURNEY

LEARN THROUGH ACTIVITY

1. Please come up with a research question and study goal related to a topic of interest that could best be answered with a mixed methods research design. Which mixed methods study would be most appropriate for your goals? Which data type would you prioritize and why?
2. Read one of the mixed methods design studies that was referenced in Table 8-3 and identify the sampling strategies utilized by the authors. Additionally, identify which type of data was prioritized and then reflect on whether this was the best approach given the purpose of goals of the study.

CHECK YOUR KNOWLEDGE

1. If a mixed methods study was prioritizing the qualitative data, which lettering system would be used to indicate this priority?

   a. QUAL

   b. qual

   c. QUAN

   d. quan

2. Some researchers believe that mixed methods research design is not appropriate because qualitative and quantitative data are seen as incompatible. What did Reichardt and Rallis refer to this viewpoint as?

   a. Postpositivist worldview

   b. Pragmatist theory

   c. Paradigm debate

   d. Convergent paradigm

3. Mixed methods research design sampling uses a combination of probability and purposive sampling.

   a. True

   b. False

4. Although there are many benefits to mixed methods research designs, some weaknesses are inherent to this type of research. Which of the following would be an identified weakness?

   a. Resolving discrepancies that arise between different types of data

   b. The time required to collect and analyze data

   c. The opportunity to collaborate with a wide variety of researchers

   d. a and b

5. If the goal of a research study is the development of a new instrument and qualitative data are collected and analyzed first, followed by quantitative data, which study design is this describing?

   a. Sequential exploratory

   b. Embedded

   c. Sequential explanatory

   d. Multiphase

6. Before conducting a mixed methods research design study, which of the following decisions should be made?

   a. Deciding which method will take priority during data collection and analysis

   b. Determining implementation of data collection

   c. Determining if a theoretical perspective will be used

   d. All of the above

THINK ABOUT IT

1. You are planning a research study in which your goal is to cross-validate data. Specifically, you want to determine the difference in exercise habits, compliance, and attitudes toward at-home fall prevention programs between elderly patients living alone and those who live with a spouse or partner. Which mixed methods study design would be most appropriate in this situation?

2. You have decided that a mixed methods research design will be the optimal method to answer your research question examining burnout among medical residents. You reach out to a colleague to collaborate with you on this project, and she tells you that qualitative and quantitative data cannot be combined in one study. She goes on to state that certain methods just don't go together. How would you respond to this colleague to highlight the benefits of mixed methods research designs?

MAKE A STRETCH

If you are interested in conducting your own mixed method design research studies, the following resources may prove insightful.

- The Mixed Methods Research Association (http://mmira.wildapricot.org) sponsors international and regional conferences.

- The Center for Innovation in Research and Teaching (https://cirt.gcu.edu/research /developmentresources/research_ready/mixed_methods/overview) provides an overview of mixed methods research and helpful links to assist researchers in planning their own studies. Additionally, numerous peer-reviewed journals publish mixed methods research studies, including the *Journal of Mixed Methods Research*, which "focuses on empirical, methodological, and theoretical articles about mixed methods research across the social, behavioral, health, and human sciences" (http://journals .sagepub.com/home/mmr). *Field Methods* (http://journals.sagepub.com/home/fmx) "publishes articles about methods used by field investigators from the social and behavioral sciences in the collection, management, analysis and presentation of data about human thought and/or human behavior in the natural world."

REFERENCES

1. Fawcett J. Invisible nursing research: thoughts about mixed methods research and nursing practice. *Nurs Sci Q.* 2015;28(2):167-168.
2. Creswell JW, Plano Clark VL, Gutmann ML, Hanson WE. Advanced mixed methods research designs. In Tashakkori A, Teddlie C, eds. *Handbook of Mixed Methods in Social and Behavioral Research.* Thousand Oaks, CA: Sage; 2003:209-240.
3. Morse JM. Approaches to qualitative-quantitative methodological triangulation. *Nurs Res.* 1991;40:120-123.
4. Morse JM. Principles of mixed methods and multimethod research design. In Tashakkori A, Teddlie C, eds. *Handbook of Mixed Methods in Social and Behavioral Research.* Thousand Oaks, CA: Sage; 2003:189-208.
5. Campbell DT, Fiske D. Convergent and discriminant validation by the multitrait multimethod matrix. *Psychol Bull.* 1959;56:81-105.

6. Reichardt CS, Cook TD. Beyond qualitative versus quantitative methods. In Cook TD, Reichardt CS, eds. *Qualitative and Quantitative Methods in Evaluation Research*. Beverly Hills, CA: Sage; 1979:7-32.

7. Reichardt CS, Rallis SF. *The Qualitative-Quantitative Debate: New Perspectives*. San Francisco, CA: Jossey-Bass; 1994.

8. Greene JC, Caracelli VJ. Making paradigmatic sense of mixed methods practice. In Tashakkori A, Teddlie C, eds. *Handbook of Mixed Methods in Social and Behavioral Research*. Thousand Oaks, CA: Sage; 2003:91-110.

9. Rossman GB, Wilson BL. Numbers and words: combining quantitative and qualitative methods in a single large-scale evaluation study. *Eval Rev*. 1985;9:627-643.

10. Cherryholmes CC. Notes on pragmatism and scientific realism. *Educ Res* 1992;21:13-17.

11. Newman I, Ridenour CS, Newman C, DeMarco GMP, Jr. A typology of research purposes and its relationship to mixed methods. In Tashakkori A, Teddlie C, eds. *Handbook of Mixed Methods in Social and Behavioral Research*. Thousand Oaks, CA: Sage; 2003:167-188.

12. Greene JC, Caracelli VJ, Graham WF. Toward a conceptual framework for mixed-method evaluation design. *Educ Eval Policy Anal*. 1989;11:255-274.

13. Punch KF. *Introduction to Social Research: Quantitative and Qualitative Approaches*. Thousand Oaks, CA: Sage; 1998.

14. Mertens DM. Mixed methods and the politics of human research: the transformative-emancipatory perspective. In Tashakkori A, Teddlie C, eds. *Handbook of Mixed Methods in Social and Behavioral Science*. Thousand Oaks, CA: Sage; 2003:135-164.

15. Creswell JW. *A Concise Introduction to Mixed Methods Research*. Thousand Oaks, CA: Sage; 2015.

16. Creswell JW, Plano Clark VL. *Designing and Conducting Mixed Methods Research*. 2nd ed. Thousand Oaks, CA: Sage; 2011.

17. Creswell JW. *Research Design: Quantitative, Qualitative, and Mixed Methods Approaches*. 2nd ed. Thousand Oaks, CA: Sage; 2003.

18. Morgan DL. Practical strategies for combining qualitative and quantitative methods: applications to health research. *Qual Health Res*. 1998;8:362-376.

19. Hanson WE, Creswell JW, Plano Clark VL, Petski KS, Creswell JD. Mixed methods research designs in counseling psychology. *J Couns Psychol*. 2005;52(2):22-235.

20. Teddlie C, Tashakkori A. *Foundations of Mixed Methods Research: Integrating Quantitative and Qualitative Approaches in the Social and Behavioral Sciences*. Thousand Oaks, CA: Sage; 2009.

21. Creswell JW, Plano Clark VL. *Designing and Conducting Mixed Methods Research*. Thousand Oaks, CA: Sage; 2007.

22. Bishop FL. Using mixed methods research in health psychology: an illustrated discussion from a pragmatist perspective. *Br J Clin Psychol*. 2015;20:5-20.

23. Fawcett J. Thoughts about multidisciplinary, interdisciplinary, and transdisciplinary research. *Nurs Sci Q*. 2013;26:376-379.

24. Fawcett J. Thoughts about collaboration—or is it capitulation? *Nurs Sci Q*. 2014;27:260-261.

25. Zoellner J, Harris JE. Mixed-methods research in nutrition and dietetics. *J Acad Nutr Diet*. 2017;117(5):683-697.

26. Glogowska M. Paradigms, pragmatism and possibilities: mixed-methods research in speech and language therapy. *Int J Lang Commun Disord*. 2011;46(3):251-260.

27. McManamny T, Sheen J, Boyd L, Jennings PA. Mixed methods and its application in prehospital research: a systematic review. *J Mix Methods Res*. 2014;9(3):214-231.

28. Rauscher L, Greenfield BH. Advancements in contemporary physical therapy research: use of mixed methods designs. *Phys Ther*. 2009;89(1):91-100.

29. Mazerolle SM, Eason CM, Goodman A. Organizational infrastructure in the collegiate athletic training setting, part I: quality-of-life comparisons and commonalities among the models. *J Athl Train*. 2017;52(1):12-22.

30. Ashton LM, Morgan PJ, Hutchesson MJ, Rollo ME, Collins CE. Young men's preferences for design and delivery of physical activity and nutrition interventions: a mixed-methods study. *Am J Men's Health*. 2017;11(5):1588-1599.

31. De Meester K, Van Bogaert V, Clarke SP, Bossaert L. In-hospital mortality after serious adverse events on medical and surgical nursing units: a mixed methods study. *J Clin Nurs*. 2012;22:2308-2317.

32. Clement D, Granquist MD, Arvinen-Barrow M. Psychosocial aspects of athletic injuries as perceived by athletic trainers. *J Athl Train* 2013;48(4):512-521.

33. Burgermaster M, Koroly J, Contento I, Koch P, Gray HL. A mixed-methods comparison of classroom context during food, health, and choices: a childhood obesity prevention intervention. *J Sch Health.* 2017;87(11):811-822.

34. Craft J, Christensen M, Bakon S, Wirihana L. Advancing student nurse knowledge of the biomedical science: a mixed methods study. *Nurse Educ.* 2017;48:114-119.

35. Lamont S, Brunero S, Lyon S, Foster K, Perry L. Collaboration amongst clinical nursing leadership teams: a mixed-methods sequential explanatory study. *J Nurs Manag.* 2015;23:1126-1136.

36. Leggott KT, Martin M, Sklar D, et al. Transformation of anesthesia for ambulatory orthopedic surgery: a mixed-methods study of a diffusion of innovation in healthcare. *Healthcare.* 2016;4:181-187.

37. Comer C, Glover J, Richardson J, et al. Stratification of treatment in a community-based musculo-skeletal service: a mixed-methods study to assess predictors of requiring complex care. *Arch Phys Med Rehabil.* 2016;97:900-911.

38. Hebesberger D, Dondrup C, Koertner T, Gisinger C, Pripfl J. Lessons learned from the deployment of a long-term autonomous robot as companion in physical therapy for older adults with dementia: a mixed methods study. In: *The Eleventh ACM/IEEE International Conference on Human-Robot Interaction.* Christchurch, New Zealand: 2016:27-34.

39. Van den Bruel A, Jones C, Thompson M, Mant D. C-reactive protein point-of-care testing in acutely ill children: a mixed methods study in primary care. *Arch Dis Child.* 2016;101:382-386.

Being a Good Consumer of Qualitative Research

LEARNING OBJECTIVES

Readers will be able to do the following:
1. Explain the importance of evaluating qualitative research.
2. Select an appropriate set of evaluation questions to critically appraise a study.
3. Conduct a thorough and fair evaluation of a qualitative research study.

EVALUATING RESEARCH

When reviewing and reading qualitative research, it is important to understand the criteria for "good qualitative research."[1] The details shared by the researcher should be rich and comprehensive so as to ensure full disclosure and understanding of the process undertaken to answer the research aims. Cohen and Crabtree[1] suggest 7 criteria for good qualitative research: (1) carrying out ethical research, (2) importance of the topic/research, (3) clarity and coherence of the research report, (4) use of appropriate and rigorous methods, (5) importance of the reflexivity or attending to research bias, (6) importance of establishing credibility, and (7) importance of verification.

The qualitative research community currently has multiple standards for evaluating research that differs according to academic discipline, perspective, and methodology.[2] It is beyond the scope of this chapter to examine each of these in detail, but at the end we provide a list of resources for you to delve into this area of discussion and debate (called *criteriology*—yes really!) should you so choose. For now, suffice it to say that qualitative

Pitney WA, Parker J, Mazerolle Singe S, Potteiger K.
Qualitative Research in the Health Professions (pp 125-136).
© 2020 Taylor & Francis Group.

research is evaluated using a variety of standards, which differ according to academic discipline, methodology, and perspective. This chapter will help you use appropriate criteria in thoroughly and fairly evaluating qualitative research.

Significance of the Evaluation Process

It is incumbent on us as health professionals to base our decisions and actions on findings from sound research. Indeed, poor study design may result in inappropriate application of research findings when making health care decisions or creating policy.[3] In sum, when examining the findings of a qualitative research study, we want to be sure it is methodologically appropriate to have arrived at the results presented. There are several reasons for evaluating a qualitative study.

?

Why do I need to evaluate a study when writing a literature review? Could I just include the information?

When writing a review, it is best to be a critical consumer and demonstrate your understanding of the topic by discussing the content and quality of the information presented in the article.

When evaluating a qualitative research study, your goal is to determine whether the study in question has been conducted appropriately and rigorously enough to support the findings. For example, you may come across a study with findings that strongly support the importance of an investigation you are proposing. But what if the study you are reading has flaws in design or analysis that cause you to question the results? Or what if the authors have left out critical information? How will issues such as these affect your use of the study?

Like an investigative reporter, your role is to dissect the study to see whether the critical components are all present and cohesive. The critical difference between recording and evaluating is one of judgment. When you examine information from an article, you outline what you know about the study. Evaluation often begins with the question, "What do you wish you knew about this study?" In other words, what are the missing pieces? In this context, the missing pieces may be either concrete, such as detailed demographics of the participants, or conceptual, such as how the authors reached their conclusions based on the results. Remember, good research often generates more questions than it answers, but the questions should be related to a future study rather than the current article.

Developing an Impartial Evaluative Lens

It is important to have an open mind when reviewing the literature and to focus on the content and details provided within the manuscript. Just as the researchers must remove, yet still address, their biases in the manuscript, you as the consumer of the product must be aware of your own personal and professional biases. It is important to review the purpose and goal of the study and then determine whether the process shared provides credibility and rigor. Can you believe the researchers? Although there is some flexibility within the qualitative research paradigm, rich information should be shared to provide the reader with the ability to believe the findings and see how the study was carried out, as well as how those findings answer the research questions and purpose.

As you begin your evaluation, remember that the authors invested time and energy in the process of qualitative research and did not deliberately set out to confuse you. This comment may seem a little flippant, but our intent is to encourage you to approach evaluation with respect for the authors and the process. Think of evaluation as an educational opportunity rather than a negative experience. Evaluating the article will not only assist you in your assignments, it will also help you strengthen your own writing. Just as reviewing the literature helps you develop study proposals, evaluating articles helps you determine what works for you as both a reader and a writer.

I do not mean to be pejorative, but the study I am evaluating seems pathetic. What should I do?

Pathetic is a very strong word. Use it cautiously! You may need to change your evaluative lens for this particular study. Think about how the process of learning from the author's mistakes strengthens your own research skills. If you are required to give feedback to this author, you can always find something positive. It may be their willingness to submit their work for critical evaluation (which takes courage) or the nature of the topic itself.

Remember that the content of an article is often at the mercy of journal format, page restrictions, and journal reviewers. If you need additional information, rather than mentally scolding the authors for their lack of detail, consider personally contacting them to ask for clarification. This bold move serves 2 key purposes: you will both obtain the information you need for your own research and establish contact with a researcher who shares your interests or methodology. Congratulations—you have just begun to develop your research network!

Finally, try to remove any bias about a particular topic or researcher from your evaluation. Just as authors must disclose their biases and research connections, so must you—your evaluation lens must be clear. For example, if you have strongly held beliefs about stem cell research, can you fairly evaluate a study that investigates this topic? Further, if you have read several articles by the same author and do not particularly like her style of writing or have questioned some of her past research, can you be impartial in evaluating her latest research contribution? Keep these questions in mind as you begin the evaluation process.

STARTING THE EVALUATION PROCESS

Several reasons for evaluating qualitative studies exist, so your purpose will determine the questions you ask and the time you need to devote to the process. At the most basic level, the evaluation process requires you to judge the "trustworthiness and plausibility of the researcher's account."[4] In other words, do you believe that the researchers did what they outlined in their methods section? Do you believe the findings of the study? If so, why do you believe the researchers? If not, why do you distrust them? By answering these questions, you are well on your way to becoming an evaluator.

? *My colleague and I read the same qualitative research study, and he thought it was very believable, but I do not buy the results—that is to say, the study does not seem believable to me. Am I wrong?*

Not necessarily. Remember that qualitative research is highly contextual, so your interpretation is filtered through your own experiences. The beauty and the frustration of qualitative research is that a study may resonate with your colleague but not with you.

Although these questions are certainly important, Mays and Pope[5] identified 2 goals for qualitative researchers: "to create an account of method and data which can stand independently so that another trained researcher could [analyze] the same data in the same way and come to essentially the same conclusions; and to produce a plausible and coherent explanation of the phenomenon under scrutiny." These goals can be translated into questions for evaluating a qualitative study. Namely, do you have enough information about the study's design and participants to conduct a similar study? Do the authors logically link the results to the conclusions?

As previously mentioned, qualitative researchers are themselves an integral part of the process. Therefore, when evaluating qualitative research, you must determine whether the researchers have addressed their personal connection to the context. This phenomenon is called *reflexivity*.[4] As you evaluate an article, ask yourself how the author addresses issues of reflexivity.

As you initially evaluate a qualitative research study, we suggest that you ask the following questions, which we call the *fab 5:*

1. Do you believe that the researchers did what they outlined in their methods section? Do you believe the findings are plausible?
2. Do you have enough information about the study's design and participants to conduct a similar study?
3. Do the authors make logical links between the results and conclusions sections?
4. How do the authors address issues of reflexivity?
5. Do the methods help you get to know the participants?

? *I do not believe this study, but my advisor is telling me to include it in my review of literature, which would change the rationale for my own study. What do I do?*

Search your beliefs for the answer. Ask yourself honestly whether you are discounting the study because of its flaws or because it does not support your own research agenda. If there is any truth in the latter answer, set your own agenda aside and do the right thing by including the study.

DIGGING DEEPER

If you are conducting a more thorough evaluation of a study to determine how it should be considered in your review of literature, for example, in addition to the questions listed earlier, there are others you will need to consider. The key here is to dig a little deeper into the study. To assist you, we have formulated some questions for evaluation that we call our *top 10:*

1. Does the background information in the introduction lead you logically to the problem statement? Is the research problem related to the purpose statement?
2. Do the authors clearly articulate the study's conceptual framework? Does the literature review support the need for the current study?
3. Have the authors clarified their stance, bias, and experience with the topic under investigation?
4. Do the authors clearly describe the participants and how they were selected?
5. Do the authors fully describe their procedures for data collection and analysis? Are the procedures appropriate for this study?
6. Do the researchers directly and appropriately address issues of trustworthiness?
7. Do the authors present the results clearly and support them with quotes and descriptions?
8. Do the authors compare the key findings of the study with those from existing literature?
9. Are the conclusions logically based on the data presented?
10. Do the authors adequately address the study's limitations?

As you can see from the list, these questions build on our fab 5 and provide more guidance for conducting your evaluation. However, they may make you ask, "How many times can I answer no to the preceding questions before deciding to discard a particular study?" Fowkes and Fulton[6] answer this question well when they say, "Unfortunately, there is no magical formula which will convert assessments of details into an overall score on the worth of a paper." When in doubt, return to the first question of the fab 5. If you truly do not believe the results and have substantive evidence that supports your perspective, you may need to exclude the article from your literature review. However, attach your notes to the article, keep it in your files, and be prepared to explain your decision.

CONDUCTING A FULL REVIEW

Conducting a full review of a manuscript is not a task to be taken lightly. A detailed review can take many hours. Begin by reading the manuscript all the way through, just as the authors intended. This practice serves 2 key purposes. First, it gives you an overall sense of the paper. The authors deliberately structured their article or manuscript in a particular manner, and you should respect their choice. Second, this process saves you time in the long run. When we were first-time reviewers, we sat down with a list of evaluation questions and filled them out as we read the paper. Although this approach may sound logical, it was often frustrating. We would spend lots of time giving extensive feedback on a piece of information we thought was missing, only to find that very piece of information in a place we had not anticipated. However, it was located exactly where the authors intended. If we had read the entire manuscript, we would have known!

After reading the entire article or manuscript, you must ask some pointed questions. Several authors provide detailed lists for readers to consider when critically evaluating a research report. They include questions related to content (the research itself) and questions related to writing (how the research is presented). We have drawn from the work of Creswell[2]; Locke, Silverman, and Spirduso[7]; McMillan and Wergin[8]; and Merriam[9] to create a list of questions that we call our *thought-provoking 34*. We hope they will guide you through even the most detailed evaluations.

Title and Abstract

1. Does the title indicate important constructs and relationships from the study?
2. Does the abstract provide enough information to help readers decide whether to examine the full report?
3. After reading the title, abstract, and statement of purpose, are you interested in reading the next part of the study?

Introduction

4. Do the authors introduce the topic of the study in terms of previous investigations?
5. Do the authors sufficiently explain how the study fits into the present body of knowledge?
6. Is the purpose of the study clearly stated? Does the introductory material make it easy to locate?
7. If the relevant literature contains conflicting findings, did the authors discuss them?
8. Do the references include articles that have been peer-reviewed and published in the last 5 years?
9. Do the authors clearly define unique terms?
10. Do the researchers provide a balanced view of the problem and make their assumptions clear in the introduction?

Participants

11. Do the authors fully describe the participants?
12. Do the authors fully explain the sampling strategies?
13. Do the authors describe where they observed or interviewed the participants?
14. Do the authors describe why they chose the participants? Do they explain any limitations or potential biases that affected the selection process?
15. Is there evidence that the authors treated participants according to ethical standards?
16. Have the authors explained why the number of participants is appropriate for the study's procedures and purposes?

Methods

17. Do the authors identify and explain the study's design?
18. Do they rationalize their design selection?
19. Do they explain their decisions about the study's design and procedures in terms of the effectiveness or ineffectiveness of previous investigations?

20. Do the authors name and describe all the processes of data collection and analysis used in the study?
21. Do they clearly address trustworthiness by employing several different strategies?
22. Do they articulate the environmental conditions in which they collected data?
23. Do the authors indicate which protocol they used for each data collection and analysis procedures?
24. Do they clearly identify their timeline for the study and data collection and analysis procedures?
25. Do they articulate how they recorded their data?

Results and Discussion Sections

26. Do the authors clearly report the study's findings?
27. Do they clearly link the findings to the original research questions?
28. Do the titles of the emergent themes capture the essence of the data? Are the themes supported with direct participant quotes?
29. If present, do the figures and tables enhance your understanding of the study?
30. Do the titles and captions accurately represent the content of the figures and tables?
31. Are the authors' conclusions in line with the findings, or do they veer into unsupported speculation?
32. Do the authors explain how the study's results fit into the existing base of knowledge?
33. Do the authors thoroughly present the study's limitations?
34. Have the authors adequately answered the question, "So what?"

Many journals provide reviewing guidelines with sections for evaluators to complete, but these sections are often broad and correspond to the components of an article (ie, introduction, method, results, and discussion). However, the questions from the thought-provoking 34 serve 2 roles. They help us make decisions about the manuscript, and they lead us to evidence that supports our decision. From there, we can generate specific feedback for the authors.

Published Guidelines for Reviewing Qualitative Research: Consolidated Criteria for Reporting Qualitative Research

Tong, Sainsbury, and Craig[3] developed criteria for reporting qualitative research with a 32-item checklist (Consolidated Criteria for Reporting Qualitative Research [COREQ]). The checklist includes 3 major sections: (1) research team and reflexivity, (2) study design, and (3) analysis and findings. The checklist of items was designed to help researchers generate a report that provides rich details regarding the study and to help create rigor within manuscripts using a qualitative paradigm.

Research Team and Reflexivity

The first domain is defined by 2 components: *personal characteristics* and *the researcher's relationship with the participants*. Information pertaining to the researcher should be provided within the research manuscript, and this often includes the roles of each researcher and any background information that can serve as educational to the reader. Tong, Sainsbury, and Craig[3] suggest information such as who completed the interviews can be valuable information for the reader, and thus details such as years of experience/ training, credentials, and occupation of the researcher should be provided in the manuscript. Additionally, the relationship with the participants should be described, including how the relationship was formed, what the participants knew about the researcher, and why the research was being conducted.

Study Design

The second domain as described by Tong, Sainsbury, and Craig[3] includes a discussion of the *theoretical framework*, *participation selection and recruitment*, *the setting, data, and the collection process*. Researchers should provide a summation of the methodological orientation used to ground the study (eg, grounded theory, ethnography) and some rationale behind its selection. Details regarding the methods of sampling (eg, purposive), sample size (discussion of saturation should be also included), and how participants were recruited should be discussed. Specifics should be included on inclusion and exclusion criteria, and sufficient information on the participants who completed the study should be provided to ensure they met the criteria outlined.

Analysis and Findings

The final domain is focused on how the data were coded and the findings that emerge after the coding process is completed. Specifically, there should be a focus on the analysis process, as well as the steps used to establish credibility and trustworthiness.[3] As a general rule, authors should describe the analysis process in great detail and include a minimum of 2 trustworthiness strategies.[10]

Although guidelines are often offered by journals, it is important to have an established set of criteria to guide the peer review process. Like quantitative research, qualitative studies must be thoroughly evaluated to establish the rigor, integrity, and worth of the research. Think of the evaluation process as a target in which the questions from the fab 5 are the primary target, with the more specific guidelines and criteria as a metric used to provide a comprehensive review.

? **There are so many evaluation questions and so little time! Is there a shortcut for conducting a manuscript evaluation for a journal?**

No! If you do not have enough time to thoroughly evaluate a manuscript, you should politely decline the invitation to review it. Remember the quality of your review directly influences the quality of the publication and your reputation as a reviewer.

EVALUATING SPECIFIC TYPES OF QUALITATIVE RESEARCH

The earlier section provided 3 sets of questions to guide you through the evaluation process of general, interpretive qualitative research. In Chapter 7 you learned about other forms of qualitative research: grounded theory, ethnography, and phenomenology. If the research report you are evaluating uses one of these specific approaches, you may need to ask additional questions. Before you read the next sections, remind yourself of the critical elements of each approach. These elements will drive the evaluation questions.

Grounded Theory

When evaluating a grounded theory study, look for a clearly defined link between the themes of the data and the theoretical model presented. If either component or the link itself is missing, you should question the study. Creswell[2] suggests that a figure or diagrammatic representation of the theory should also be present in the article. Combined, these 2 ideas may be expressed in the following evaluation questions:

1. Do the authors clearly articulate the connection between emergent data categories and the theoretical model?
2. Is the theoretical model explained with both text and graphics?

Ethnography

An ethnography focuses on developing an understanding of an entire culture or cultural group. Therefore, ethnographers immerse themselves in other cultures for extended periods. When evaluating an ethnographic study, ask yourself, "Did the researcher spend enough time immersed in the culture to provide a rich description and interpretation?"

Phenomenology

The challenge of a phenomenological study is to describe the essence of a common experience. The researcher must describe the experience and what it means. When evaluating a phenomenological study, ask yourself whether the authors convey the overall experiences of the participants and describe the experience and the context.[2]

SUMMARY

Before it can claim a place in the research community, a qualitative study must be fairly evaluated to determine its rigor and plausibility. This chapter outlines 3 layers of the evaluation process. Your starting point depends on your reason for evaluating a qualitative study. Finally, this chapter provides some questions for you to consider if the study you are evaluating is a grounded theory, ethnography, or a phenomenology study.

CONTINUE YOUR EDUCATIONAL JOURNEY

LEARN THROUGH ACTIVITY

1. Cohen and Crabtree[1] present 7 criteria for good qualitative research. What components of their criteria are captured in the fab 5, top 10, or thought-provoking 34?
2. Examine the COREQ at https://academic.oup.com/intqhc/article/19/6/349/1791966. Compare and contrast this 32-item checklist with the thought-provoking 34. What is similar and different?

CHECK YOUR KNOWLEDGE

1. The debate about whether consistent and common criteria should exist for evaluating qualitative research is called:
   a. Criteriology
   b. Terminology
   c. Phenomenology
   d. Radiology
   e. Evaluometrics
2. At the most basic level, when evaluating a manuscript, you must pass judgment on which of the following aspects?
   a. Trustworthiness
   b. Plausibility of the researcher's account
   c. Length of the manuscript
   d. a and b
3. This term denotes whether researchers have disclosed their biases and personal connections with a topic of study:
   a. Reflexology
   b. Reflexivity
   c. Self-disclosure
   d. a and c
   e. a and b

4. When conducting a full manuscript review, your first step should be to:
   a. Provide feedback on the introduction
   b. Read the entire manuscript
   c. Give specific feedback on the methods
   d. Make an initial judgment of the topic's importance to you
   e. a and b

5. When reviewing this form of research, you must determine whether the researcher has spent enough time immersed in the culture:
   a. Ethnography
   b. Grounded theory
   c. Phenomenology
   d. a and c
   e. a and b

6. Which of the following should be clearly identified in the manuscript of a grounded theory study?
   a. Cultural description
   b. Graphic image with a timeline for the study
   c. Exhaustive description of the phenomenon
   d. Theoretic model
   e. a and b

THINK ABOUT IT

1. You have been asked by a journal to conduct a blind review of a manuscript, but you can identify the author by its title. How would handle this situation?

2. A colleague is very upset by a review she received for her manuscript and asks for your opinion. When you read the review, you realize that you wrote it. How should you proceed?

3. You are angry because you do not agree with the committee's evaluation of your thesis draft. You plan to either write a scathing response or call a committee meeting. Is this your best choice of action? What other options might you have?

MAKE A STRETCH

The following resources provide an interesting dialogue on some of the issues associated with evaluating qualitative research:

- Anderson C. Presenting and evaluating qualitative research. *Am J Pharm Educ.* 2010;74(8):141.
- Kitto SC, Chesters J, Grbich C. Quality in qualitative research. *Med J Aust.* 2008;188(4):243-246.
- Pickler RH. Evaluating qualitative research studies. *J Pediatr Health Care.* 2007;21:195-197.

- Reynolds J, Kizito J, Ezumah N, et al. Quality assurance of qualitative research: a review of the discourse. *Health Res Policy Syst.* 2001;9, 43.
- Wu S, Wyant DC, Fraser MW. Author guidelines for manuscripts reporting on qualitative research. *J Soc Social Work Res.* 2016;7(2):405-425. [This article provides a particularly thorough set of guidelines for the reporting of qualitative research.]

REFERENCES

1. Cohen DJ, Crabtree BF. Evaluative criteria for qualitative research in health care: controversies and recommendations. *Annals Fam Med.* 2008;6(4):331-339.
2. Creswell JW. *Qualitative Inquiry & Research Design: Choosing Among Five Approaches.* 2nd ed. Thousand Oaks, CA: Sage; 2007.
3. Tong A, Sainsbury P, Craig J. Consolidated criteria for reporting qualitative research (COREQ): a 32-item checklist for interviews and focus groups. *Int J Qual Health Care.* 2007;19(6):349-357.
4. Horsburgh D. Evaluation of qualitative research. *J Clin Nurs.* 2003;12:307-312.
5. Mays N, Pope C. Qualitative research: rigour and qualitative research. *BMJ.* 1995;311:109-112.
6. Fowkes FGR, Fulton PM. Critical appraisal of published research: introductory guidelines. *BMJ.* 1991;302:1136-1140.
7. Locke LF, Silverman SJ, Spirduso WW. *Reading and Understanding Research.* Thousand Oaks, CA: Sage 1998.
8. McMillan J, Wergin J. *Understanding and Evaluating Educational Research.* 2nd ed. Upper Saddle River, NJ: Merrill; 2002.
9. Merriam SB, ed. *Qualitative Research in Practice: Examples for Discussion and Analysis.* San Francisco, CA: Jossey-Bass; 2002.
10. Creswell JW. *Qualitative Inquiry and Research Design: Choosing Among Five Approaches.* 3rd ed. Washington, DC: Sage; 2013.

Qualitative Research in Evidence-Based Practice

Readers will be able to do the following:
1. Integrate the use of qualitative evidence into the traditional 5-step approach to evidence-based practice (EBP).
2. Evaluate qualitative research for methodological rigor.
3. Describe how qualitative methods may inform clinical decisions.

EVIDENCE-BASED PRACTICE

In 1981 the *Canadian Medical Association Journal* published a series of articles aimed at teaching clinicians how to incorporate the findings of published research into their daily practice. The purpose of these publications was to help busy clinicians, mainly physicians, efficiently and effectively locate, read, and evaluate the findings of recently published studies so their clinical practice could remain consistent with valid, new knowledge.[1] This series of articles was a catalyst for change that evolved into the modern-day health care initiative of EBP.

EBP is a 5-step approach (Figure 10-1) that encourages the use of the best available evidence; the clinician's expertise; and the patient's unique characteristics, values, and/or circumstances to inform care.[2] These 3 facets are sometimes referred to as the 3-legged stool of EBP (Figure 10-2).[3] The aim of this chapter is to provide a guide for incorporating the methods of qualitative inquiry into each of the 3 aspects of EBP.

Pitney WA, Parker J, Mazerolle Singe S, Potteiger K.
Qualitative Research in the Health Professions (pp 137-147).
© 2020 Taylor & Francis Group.

Figure 10-1. The 5-step approach to EBP.

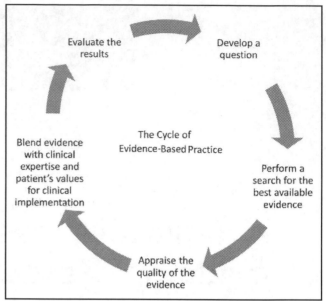

Figure 10-2. The 3-legged stool of EBP.

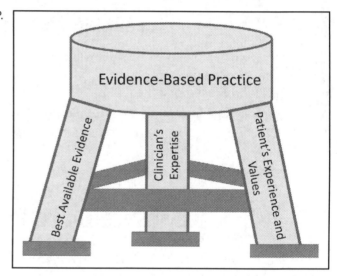

Role of Qualitative Research in Evidence-Based Practice

Most clinicians assume the evidence used in EBP must be knowledge generated from experimental research. It is even suggested by Sackett's Levels of Evidence and Grades of Recommendation, which rates nonexperimental evidence as level 5, or the lowest level of evidence.[4] However, Sackett's classification of evidence was developed to guide clinicians through a clinical question related to medication therapy for a specific condition.[5] It does not seem that Sackett even intended his rules to apply to all evidence, for he said, "Evidence-based medicine is not restricted to randomized trials and meta-analyses. It involves tracing down the best external evidence with which to answer our clinical questions."[5(p72)] Experimental research is not free of problems. It may be poor quality, difficult to evaluate, or not directly relevant to patient care.[6] It is important to remember that knowledge comes in all forms. Practice issues can be complex, and no single type of evidence in isolation can or should inform practice. Additionally, not all questions can be answered through quantitative methods, and a strict adherence to a particular research paradigm may allow important details to be missed.[6]

Qualitative research is different from quantitative studies in 3 distinct areas: (1) agenda, (2) anatomy, and (3) autonomy.[7] The agenda, or purpose, of qualitative studies focuses on the humanistic or behavioral aspects (ie, perceptions) of clinical care, whereas quantitative studies tend to focus on the biological or physiological aspects (ie, efficacy of treatment); however, both aspects are important for improved patient care. Because the agenda is different, the anatomy of qualitative research must also be different. The results of qualitative inquiry are contextualized, rich, and dense. In other words, a qualitative study's findings are often voluminous, complex, and relate specifically to a participant's own circumstances. This allows the reader an in-depth understanding of the participant's viewpoint. Due to their intricate nature, decision makers may perceive qualitative research as too cumbersome to undertake and/or use in their clinical findings. However, it is the level of detail, or degree of subjectivity, that provides the usefulness of the information. When the degree of subjectivity is understood, the reader can feel confident that the data are strong enough to stand on their own merit. The degree of subjectivity of data can be divided into 3 types[7]:

1. *Direct data*: These data are actual and concrete. By definition, this type of data is often known and is not the most enlightening. It is important that research using this type of data represents the participants exactly. Therefore, methods of verification are of utmost importance.

2. *Semidirect data*: These data are collected in the form of perceptions and emotions. By nature, this type is not concrete and is subjective. These data are subject to error and are not as concrete as direct data. However, a participant's perceptions of events are valid, even if not grounded in fact. These data provide insight into why subjects believe or act as they do.

3. *Indirect data*: These data are considered inferential and consist of subtleties, such as signs, signals, or symbols, rather than direct dialogue. Therefore, they are most susceptible to error. However, it is analysis of this type of data that often leads to innovation. When using this type of data, verification is no longer needed and may invalidate the analysis. Instead, having insight into the research process, knowledge of the literature, and immersion in the data allows for interpretation and provides an authority of analysis.

Each type of data form varies in appropriateness of qualitative design. For instance, phenomenological studies rely on direct data, whereas ethnography tends to rely on more indirect data sources.

Finally, qualitative evidence is autonomous. There are some instances in which the role of qualitative inquiry is to guide or add value to quantitative inquiry. This is often referred to as a *mixed methods approach*. Qualitative methods should also be able to stand alone on their own merit. Most studies are small and narrowly focused by design. This can limit the generalizability of findings, but it may be possible to recontextualize the research findings to similar situations. However, you must first evaluate the research to ensure it is of reasonable scope, conducted rigorously, and developed theoretically so that the findings may stand on their own.

? *What does recontextualize mean?*

Recontextualize means to see something in a different light. When reading a research article, it is helpful to consider the circumstances (ie, context) surrounding the original study and how the environment may have influenced the findings. Often, you can gain a sense of the context through the introduction or methods section. By doing this, you can better determine if the study's findings may apply to your own situation.

EVALUATING THE RESEARCH

The first leg of the stool is to use the best available evidence; after all, it is what differentiates EBP from "regular" clinical practice. Although the evidence may receive top billing, it is not the end-all-be-all. The reader must be careful in selection, evaluation, and application to ensure the evidence applies to the individual patient, as well as how it should be integrated into a clinical decision.[4] When selecting the evidence, it is important that it carries the weight of authority. Unlike our quantitative counterparts, there is not a popular method of appraisal or classification instrument to evaluate the quality of evidence. Therefore, it is up to the qualitative research community to develop a guide for users to appropriately appraise and classify their evidence. Several researchers have done so; however, none have emerged as the clear-cut favorite.[8] Therefore, we present the Decision Rules for Incorporating Qualitative Research in EBP accompanied by the Rosalind Franklin-Qualitative Research Appraisal Instrument (RF-QRA).[9]

Appraising the Literature

Henderson and Rheault's[9] Decision Rules for Incorporating Qualitative Research used in conjunction with the RF-QRA provides a means to evaluate the methodological rigor of qualitative studies that mirrors Sackett's Levels of Evidence and Grades of Recommendations. These instruments were developed to serve as a guide for clinicians to incorporate qualitative research into the EBP framework.

There are 4 questions for the reader to consider when determining if a qualitative study should be used in answering their clinical question. They are:

1. Is the research study peer reviewed?
2. Does the study seek to describe a social or human issue in a natural setting through either in-depth interviews or observations?
3. Does the study provide an interpretation of data that goes beyond simple description?
4. Did the authors adhere to qualitative research ethics?

If the study passes the initial screen, the clinician should use the RF-QRA (Figure 10-3) to assess the study's methodological rigor and determine the study's level of evidence (Table 10-1) and grade the recommendation of the body of evidence (Table 10-2). These decision rules, combined with the RF-QRA, provide a quick and simple method of appraising the methodological rigor of qualitative studies, even for those with limited knowledge of qualitative methods. In terms of how to rank qualitative manuscripts on the evidence hierarchy, Henderson and Rheult provided a system similar to Sackett's; however, because the methods are so distinct, we must use a scale created specifically for qualitative inquiry.

ROSALIND FRANKLIN-QUALITATIVE RESEARCH
APPRAISAL INSTRUMENT (RF-QRA)

1. CREDIBILITY

Can you believe the results?   Credible   Relevant Problems

Example Strategies:
- Prolonged engagement
- Field journal
- Subjects judge results as credible
- Triangulation—multiple data sources,
            methods, or investigators
- Establish competence of researcher

2. TRANSFERABILITY

Can the results be transferred to other situations?   Transferable   Relevant Problems

Example Strategies:
- Detailed description of sample and context
- Compare sample to larger group
- Representative sample

3. DEPENDABILITY

Would the results be similar if the study was repeated?   Dependable   Relevant Problems

Example Strategies:
- Detailed description of methods
- Two or more researchers independently judge the data
- Triangulation—multiple data sources,
            methods, or investigators
- Code–recode procedure
- Peer examination/external audit

4. CONFIRMABILITY

Was there an attempt to enhance objectivity by
reducing research bias?   Confirmable   Relevant Problems

Example Strategies:
- Triangulation—multiple data sources,
            methods, or investigators
- External audit
- Field journal

Figure 10-3. Critically appraising qualitative inquiry. (Reprinted with permission from Henderson R, Rheault W. Appraising and incorporating qualitative research in evidence-based practice. *J Phys Ther Educ.* 2004;18[3]:35-40.)

The system that Henderson and Rheult describe is designed specifically for appraising the methodological rigor needed to ensure trustworthiness in qualitative inquiry (Figure 10-4). Because its language is consistent with that of Sackett's framework[4] for quantitative research, the RF-QRA is a familiar alternative for clinicians when evaluating qualitative studies. After the best available evidence is identified, step 4 of the EBP process is to blend the research findings with the clinician's expertise and the patient's unique characteristics, values, and/or circumstances to inform care. After all, if the evidence suggests a treatment that is unavailable to the clinician or that is inconsistent with the patient's values or circumstances, then the evidence, regardless of its methodological quality, is not useful to the clinician.

TABLE 10-1

QUALITATIVE LEVELS OF EVIDENCE

LEVEL	CRITERIA
I	Affirmative response to all 4 aspects of trustworthiness as outlined in the RF-QRA without any relevant problems
II	Affirmative responses to 3 of the 4 aspects of trustworthiness as outlined in the RF-QRA without any relevant problems and issues with 1 of the 4 aspect of trustworthiness
III	Affirmative responses to 2 of the 4 aspects of trustworthiness as outlined in the RF-QRA without any relevant problems and issues with the other 2 aspects of trustworthiness
IV	An affirmative response to 1 of the 4 aspects of trustworthiness as outlined in the RF-QRA without any relevant problems and issues with the other 3 aspects of trustworthiness
V	Relevant problems with all 4 aspects of trustworthiness as outlined in the RF-QRA

Adapted from Henderson R, Rheault W. Appraising and incorporating qualitative research in evidence-based practice. *J Phys Ther Educ.* 2004;18(3):35-40.

TABLE 10-2

QUALITATIVE GRADES OF RECOMMENDATION

GRADE	CRITERIA
A	Outcomes are supported by at least one Level I study (preferably more).
B	Outcomes are supported by at least one Level II study.
C	Outcomes are supported by at least one Level III, IV, or V study.

Adapted from Henderson R, Rheault W. Appraising and incorporating qualitative research in evidence-based practice. *J Phys Ther Educ.* 2004;18(3):35-40.

INFORMING CLINICAL DECISIONS

Qualitative inquiry does not seek to find truth, but instead seeks to acknowledge the existence and interplay of multiple views.[7] Qualitative evidence can be a powerful resource for informing clinical decisions because it can help the clinician understand how their decisions are perceived by their patients, as well as why their prescribed interventions may or may not be successful.

Qualitative methods are particularly useful for exploring how outcomes are achieved. However, the context and the impact of the specific situation or setting of the study on its findings should not be ignored.[10] Aspects such as the logistics involved, how a patient's

Decision Rules for Incorporating Qualitative Research Into Evidence-Based Practice

Decision 1: The study satisfies the general assumptions for inclusion in the review.
Assumptions
- Research studies are peer reviewed.
- Problem researched is important to the EBP question.

Decision 2: The study meets the qualitative screening criteria.
Qualitative Screens
    The inquiry process:
- Involves observation of social or human problems in the natural setting.
- Interprets observations.
- Ties observed phenomenon to understanding, explanation, or development of theory.
- Adheres to ethical principles (risk/benefit/privacy).

Decision 3: The level of qualitative evidence with the RF-QRA.
Levels of Qualitative Evidence from the RF-QRA:
Level I: Affirmative response regarding all four (4) aspects*; no relevant problem(s).
Level II: Affirmative response regarding three (3) aspects; relevant problem(s) noted in one (1) aspect.
Level III: Affirmative response regarding two (2) aspects; relevant problem(s) noted in two (2) aspects.
Level IV: Affirmative response regarding one (1) aspect; relevant problem(s) noted in three (3) aspects.
Level V: Relevant problem(s) noted in all four (4) aspects.
*Credibility, transferability, dependability, and confirmability.

Decision 4: The grade of recommendation based upon the qualitative evidence available.
Grades of Recommendation of Qualitative Evidence
Grade A: Recommendations are made for outcomes supported by at least one (1), and preferably more than one, Level I study.
Grade B: Recommendations are made for outcomes supported by at least one (1) Level II study.
Grade C: Recommendations are supported by Level III, IV, and V studies.

Figure 10-4. Determining the level and grade of evidence in qualitative inquiry. (Reprinted with permission from Henderson R, Rheault W. Appraising and incorporating qualitative research in evidence-based practice. *J Phys Ther Educ.* 2004;18[3]:35-40.)

situation may change, or motivators and barriers to treatment can provide insight as to why the implementation of an intervention was successful or not, as well as explore the decision-making processes of both practitioners and their patients. The patient's views of health and illness may be especially useful because they are often complex, internally consistent, and logical, despite sometimes being in contrast with traditional medical wisdom.

Enhancing Clinical Expertise

Clinical decisions involve determining "what is the best thing for this patient at this time?"[11] Using the EBP framework, we can reframe this question as "under these circumstances, what is the best next thing for this patient at this time?"[11(p281)] Doing so helps the clinician provide context to their patient's unique situation so there is less chance of compromising the patient's care. This leads us to our second leg of the 3-legged stool, which focuses on the clinician's expertise. Clinical expertise considers the clinician's previous experiences, clinical competence, and available resources. The process of incorporating clinical expertise can occur in many ways. One such way is for the clinician to identify relevant factors to the patient's clinical problem across the patient's life. Examples of relevant factors include but are not limited to the patient's cognitive abilities, emotional state, cultural background, spiritual beliefs, socioeconomic status, access to care, support network, work or family responsibilities, attitude regarding their illness, and their relationship with their health care providers. Failure to identify these factors can compromise the patient's outcome and is known as a *contextual error.*

Determining Patient Values

Often, health care providers and their patients have different perspectives about health and well-being. Therefore, determining "what is the best thing for the patient at this time" is not always an easy task. Consideration of the patient's characteristics and values is the final leg of the 3-legged stool. The EBP framework calls for patients and clinicians to make the best choice for "what is the best thing for this patient at this time."[12] Qualitative research may serve as a bridge between patient values and best scientific evidence.[13] It is our role as clinicians to pay careful attention to our patients' hopes, aspirations, and values.[14] In doing so, we are likely to arrive at very different treatment decisions for each patient. For example, a patient may not feel comfortable with the personal contact required for manual therapy. Therefore, even if the evidence suggests manual therapy is the best treatment option for the patient's condition, the patient may not be able to relax enough during the treatment to receive the full benefit, or the patient may not be compliant with their treatment plan. Either way, in this situation, this is not the best choice for this patient at this time.

Qualitative studies may also help practitioners better understand why individual values may lead a patient to decline a treatment even if it receives high recommendation in the literature. In their 2008 review of the literature, Micheals and colleagues[13] evaluated 2 qualitative studies in their quest to explore why 2 populations of women declined secondary prevention efforts as recommended by their health care providers. Their findings acknowledge that the decision to turn down treatment was not made in disregard to the patient's health, and patient education is not enough to reverse their decision. Instead, inviting patients to tell stories about previous medical encounters to better ascertain the patient's values and beliefs related to health, self-care, and current scientific knowledge helped the clinician better understand the patient's perspective in declining treatment. Without these types of studies, the phenomenon of saying "no" to routine medical treatment may elude clinicians and lead them to believe their patients are ambivalent about their own personal health. An understanding of these factors will help clinicians better relate to their patient population.

Finally, there are many ways of determining our patients' unique values and characteristics. We can ask questions, listen to our patients' stories, and look for subtle clues in our patient interactions. However, we must be careful to consider the role of our own personal values and how these might influence our patient interactions. One way to do this is to spend some time reflecting upon your own personal values and how they may influence your decisions—from the evidence you choose to read, to the daily decisions made during clinical practice. In doing so, you can become more aware of your personal values and how they might influence your clinical decisions. If not, you could run the risk of violating patient trust.

How do I reflect upon my own personal values?

You can do this in much the same way as if you were bracketing your biases before collecting and analyzing data. Take the time to think and write about your beliefs and values in relation to the issue at hand. Writing will help you think deeply about your beliefs.

SUMMARY

Qualitative research is an often-overlooked source of evidence in the EBP framework. This type of design can assist clinicians in answering clinical questions that experimentally driven studies cannot. No matter the design, it is important to first assess the quality of the study prior to applying it to clinical practice. However, the tools traditionally used to assess the literature were designed with experimental studies in mind and are not appropriate for evaluating observational studies. Several tools for evaluating qualitative studies are cited in the literature, including the RF-QRA Instrument and its accompanying Grades of Recommendation and Levels of Evidence, which were presented in this chapter. Once clinicians identify quality evidence, they must consider the context to determine if the findings may be generalizable. If so, they can feel comfortable blending the findings with their own clinical expertise, as well as the patient's unique characteristics and values, to guide clinical practice. However, clinicians must be careful to ensure their own personal values do not bias their decision-making process.

CONTINUE YOUR EDUCATIONAL JOURNEY

LEARN THROUGH ACTIVITY

1. Qualitative research focuses on the behavioral aspects of clinical care, whereas quantitative studies tend to focus on the biological or physiological aspects. Based on your personal experience, provide an example of a clinical question that could best be answered by qualitative research.

2. Once you have completed your clinical question, perform a search for at least one piece of qualitative evidence to answer your question. Then evaluate your evidence using the Qualitative Decision Rules and RF-QRA. Include a Level of Evidence and Grade of Recommendation as appropriate.

3. Context has been a consistent theme throughout our analysis of the 3-legged stool of EBP. Can you explain how context may affect the use of evidence as well as inform clinical decisions in your own practice?

CHECK YOUR KNOWLEDGE

1. Qualitative evidence can be evaluated for quality using the same tools as those that assess the quality of quantitative or experimental designs.
   a. True
   b. False

2. The focus of a study is known as its:
   a. Agenda
   b. Anatomy
   c. Autonomy
   d. a and b
   e. b and c

3. Which type of data is often the most insightful and can lead to innovation?
   a. Direct
   b. Semi-direct
   c. Indirect
   d. All of the above
   e. a and b

4. If a patient seems uncomfortable discussing a certain topic and changes the subject or provides short, noninformative answers when asked direct questions, what type of data would the patient's unwillingness to speak be considered?
   a. Direct data
   b. Semi-direct data
   c. Indirect data
   d. This should not be considered data because it was not verbalized

5. After recontextualizing a study, the study's findings may no longer be relevant to your clinical question.
   a. True
   b. False

THINK ABOUT IT

Your patient is a 24-year-old female who is finishing up the classroom portion of her physician's assistant professional program. She recently tore the anterior cruciate ligament in her knee and is considering undergoing reconstructive surgery. She would like to have the surgery over her holiday break prior to beginning her clinical rotations in the spring. In the attempt to avoid a contextual error, consider all of the factors that might influence your patient's outcome to determine if knee reconstruction is the best choice for the patient at this point in her life.

MAKE A STRETCH

These resources will assist you to expand your knowledge related to the EBP process, the use of qualitative evidence in EBP, and considering patient values when making clinical decisions.

- The Centre for Evidence-Based Medicine: www.cebm.net
- The Cochrane Collaboration: www.cochrane.org/
- Guyatt G, Rennie D, Meade MO, Cook DJ. *Users' Guide to the Medical Literature: Essentials of Evidence-Based Clinical Practice.* 3rd ed. New York, NY: McGraw-Hill; 2015.
- Reynolds J, Kizito J, Ezumah N, et al. Quality assurance of qualitative research: a review of the discourse. *Health Res Policy Syst.* 2011;9:43.
- Fulbrook P. Developing best practices in critical care nursing: knowledge, evidence and practice. *Nurs Crit Care.* 2003;8(3):96-102.
- Michaels C, McEwin MM, McArthur DB. Saying "no" to professional recommendations: client values, beliefs and evidence-based practice. *J Am Assoc Nurse Pract.* 2008;585-589

REFERENCES

1. How to read clinical journals, I: why to read them and how to start reading them critically. *CMAJ.* 1981;124(5):555-558.
2. Guyatt G, Rennie D, Meade MO, Cook DJ. *Users' Guide to the Medical Literature: A Manual for Evidence-Based Clinical Practice.* 2nd ed. New York, NY: McGraw-Hill; 2008.
3. Spring B. Evidence-based practice in clinical psychology: what it is, why it matters; what you need to know. *J Clin Psychol.* 2007;63(7):611-631.
4. Sackett DL, Rosenberg WM, Gray JA, Haynes RB, Richardson WS. Evidence based medicine: what it is and what it isn't. *BMJ.* 1996;312(7023):71-72.
5. Sackett DL. Rules of evidence and clinical recommendations on the use of antithrombotic agents. *Chest.* 1989;95:2S-4S.
6. Fulbrook P. Developing best practices in critical care nursing: knowledge, evidence and practice. *Nurs Crit Care.* 2003;8(3):96-102.
7. Morse JM. Reconceptualizing qualitative evidence. *Qual Health Res.* 2006;16(3):415-422.
8. Dixon-Woods M, Agarwal S, Jones D, Young B, Sutton A. Synthesizing qualitative and quantitative evidence: a review of possible methods. *J Health Serv Res Policy.* 2005;10(1):45-53.
9. Henderson R, Rheault W. Appraising and incorporating qualitative research in evidence-based practice. *J Phys Ther Educ.* 2004;18(3):35-40.
10. Barbour RS. The role of qualitative research in broadening the 'evidence base' for clinical practice. *J Eval Clin Pract.* 2000;6(2):155-163.
11. Weiner SJ. Contextualizing medical decisions to individualize care: lessons for the qualitative sciences. *J Gen Intern Med.* 2004;19:281-285.
12. Lee YK, Low WY, Ng CJ. Exploring patient values in medical decision making: a qualitative study. *PLoS One.* 2013;8(11):e80052.
13. Michaels C, McEwin MM, McArthur DB. Saying "no" to professional recommendations: client values, beliefs and evidence-based practice. *J Am Assoc Nurse Pract.* 2008;585-589
14. Kelly MP, Heath I, Howick J, Greenhalgh T. The importance of values in evidence-based medicine. *BMC Med Ethics.* 2015;16:69.

Looking Back and Moving Forward

Readers will be able to do the following:
1. Recognize and respond to arguments against qualitative research.
2. Identify practical resources for conducting qualitative research.
3. Explain principles related to creating and presenting a research proposal.

LOOKING BACK

The preceding chapters cover a great deal of information about qualitative research, including how to recognize, conceptualize, and execute a qualitative study. Our intent was to write a comprehensive text that provides practical examples from the health professions and describes the systematic processes of qualitative research in language that is easy to understand. Metaphorically, we wanted to provide a view of the forest without interference from the trees. Having read the first 10 chapters, you are ready to walk into the forest of qualitative inquiry. Our final task is to provide additional tools for your journey of conducting effective qualitative research and being a critical consumer of qualitative research findings.

You may wonder what you will need to be a successful qualitative researcher. We present 2 sets of tools to assist you. The first will help you respond professionally to frequent arguments made against qualitative research. The second will provide practical, nuts-and-bolts information about completing a qualitative study.

Pitney WA, Parker J, Mazerolle Singe S, Potteiger K.
Qualitative Research in the Health Professions (pp 149-163).
© 2020 Taylor & Francis Group.

DEFENDING YOUR QUALITATIVE RESEARCH

This section begins with 3 anecdotes that illustrate some of the biases against qualitative research that we have experienced personally. William Pitney was once asked at a job interview if he did "that touchy-feely research." Despite the fact that one of us has an undergraduate minor in mathematics, we have been asked if we are afraid of the statistics associated with quantitative research. We as qualitative researchers have also been called the junior varsity team compared to the varsity team of quantitative researchers. Although these examples are meant to provide levity, they elucidate a dominant scholarly attitude toward the interpretive research paradigm. You will likely encounter critics during your work in qualitative research, and you could easily feel defensive when articulating your position. However, emotional arguments are usually unproductive and unpersuasive. In most instances arguments and criticisms are borne from myths that are created by assumptions that are held about the interpretive research paradigm. This section outlines typical assumptions against and criticisms of qualitative research and suggests potential responses. The names of the 2 characters, Dr. Skeptic and Dr. Convincing, are deliberately chosen to signify the positions of the quantitative and qualitative researchers. You have a professional obligation to politely respond to Dr. Skeptic. However, you should not be subjected to Dr. Angry, Dr. Pejorative, or Dr. Disrespectful. When you meet Dr. Skeptic, be strong. Do not become Dr. Defensive or Dr. Emotional!

? Why are some scholars skeptical of qualitative research in light of the strong arguments supporting its value and use?

You will encounter colleagues who are only familiar with the quantitative paradigm. With such a focused approach to research, being open to and accepting alternative methods can be challenging. Our suggestion is to keep gently educating where possible and remember that change takes time, but it is always worth the wait.

Assumption 1: Qualitative Research Is Not Rigorous

Dr. Skeptic: I am really surprised that you have chosen to conduct qualitative research. It appears that you are taking the easy way out. Qualitative research is simply not rigorous.

Dr. Convincing: If you determine rigor primarily with the standards of reliability and validity, I can understand your concern. Honestly, I also feel skeptical anytime I read a study that does not address why I should trust the data presented. However, a thorough process similar to that of quantitative research exists within the interpretive paradigm called *establishing trustworthiness*. Trustworthiness is a general term that covers issues of credibility, transferability, and dependability of data. I would be happy to share specific strategies that qualitative researchers use to ensure trustworthiness with you.

Assumption 2: Qualitative Research Is Not Objective

Dr. Skeptic: Qualitative research seems so subjective and biased. Most of the data include personal perceptions of experience. Objective data are far more important, are they not?

Dr. Convincing: Some scholars prefer data that can be quantified or measured. Many disciplines require measurements to answer specific questions, such as how a medication affects specific biomarkers. However, not all research questions can be answered with measurements. This is particularly true in social sciences, which attempt to understand human relationships and experiences. Subjective data, such as beliefs, perceptions, values, and attitudes, influence how humans act and interact. The concept of subjectivity also relates to the way in which research is conducted. Aren't all research methods of data collection and analysis beholden to the decisions of the researcher? Any time a researcher makes a choice, a level of subjectivity enters the scene. All research methods have strengths and weaknesses, and you must select the approach that best suits your research question. The use of subjective information should not automatically discredit a study.

Assumption 3: Qualitative Research Is Not Scientific

Dr. Skeptic: I believe that the most important and highest form of knowledge is based in science. To me, qualitative research just seems too arbitrary and unsystematic to be considered scientific.

Dr. Convincing: To answer you, I need to refer to the work of Dingwall,[1] who succinctly states "one of the greatest methodological fallacies of the last half century in social research is the belief that science is a particular set of techniques; it is, rather, a state of mind, or attitude, and the organizational conditions which allow that attitude to be expressed." The hallmark of science is empirical, systematic inquiry to answer purposeful and important research questions. Therefore, my goal as a qualitative researcher is to gain insight and understanding through clearly articulated, systematic methods that investigate the perceptions and experiences of others.

Assumption 4: Qualitative Research Is Merely Storytelling

Dr. Skeptic: I really enjoyed the story you wrote about the experiences that physicians have in working with patients who are dealing with obesity.

Dr. Convincing: What story are you referring to?

Dr. Skeptic: The one you published in the latest issue of our journal.

Dr. Convincing: Oh, you must be referring to the qualitative research study on physicians' perceptions and stigma associated with obese patients.

Dr. Skeptic: That was research?

Dr. Convincing: Yes. A story contains several characters and a literary plot. A research study systematically collects, analyzes, and interprets data, then identifies major themes or patterns of participants' experience. The study you read presented several themes identifying physicians' perceptions of obesity. Let me clarify with the example of a standard fairy tale. If the story of the 3 little pigs were a qualitative research study, it would fully outline the participants' demographics, including the average age of the pigs and the duration of time they spent in their homes. It would also compare the location of the homes to one another and articulate whether the pigs had a previous relationship with the wolf. Data from detailed interviews would then identify the wolf's motive for destroying the homes of the first 2 pigs. You, as a researcher, might ask the question, "What process did the big bad wolf use to destroy the homes?" You would likely conduct a grounded theory study to answer that question and create a preventive theoretical model. As you can see, fundamental differences exist between a story and a qualitative research study.

Assumption 5: Qualitative Research Cannot Be Generalized

Dr. Skeptic: What good is qualitative research if I can't apply the findings to a broad population? Doesn't this difficulty in generalization substantially limit this form of study?

Dr. Convincing: The purpose of qualitative research is to gain insight and understanding, not to apply findings to a broad population. Although the findings may not be generalized, they can often be transferred to similar contexts. For optimal transferability, qualitative researchers must carefully describe the details of the context to help readers locate the findings that apply to their own situations. This technique helps qualitative research make a valuable contribution to the existing base of knowledge.

Assumption 6: Qualitative Research Cannot Be Reproduced

Dr. Skeptic: Because the findings of qualitative research cannot be reproduced, I believe they are unreliable. My research would be severely criticized if another researcher could not replicate my study and its findings.

Dr. Convincing: It is very important for quantitative researchers to be able to reproduce their findings, especially in controlled laboratory settings. However, qualitative researchers study participants in their natural settings, which vary greatly from one study to the next. The people, school, and local community may all be different. Therefore, qualitative researchers should not expect to obtain the exact same results when repeating a study. They should explain the steps of their study with enough clarity and detail that another researcher could conduct a similar investigation.

My advisor recommends taking courses in both quantitative and qualitative research, but I want to focus on the qualitative paradigm. What should I do?

Taking classes covering both research paradigms will make you a well-rounded and well-respected researcher. Moreover, we live in a world where many important health-related questions are asked, and a single research paradigm is not likely to address them all.

The preceding examples outline the role of educator that you will likely assume to help others understand qualitative research. Be prepared to provide information about the nature of qualitative research, such as how data are collected and analyzed and how trustworthiness is addressed. Because you may need to compare and contrast qualitative and quantitative research, you should also learn about the quantitative paradigm. As you speak with others and educate them about qualitative research, you might point out that each research paradigm has a different focus and addresses different problems. In many instances, the paradigms can be used together to thoroughly research a particular topic.

I have conceptualized my study and developed my purpose and research questions. I think a mixed methods approach would be the most appropriate, but I have limited knowledge of quantitative research. What should I do?

The answer to this tough question depends on your situation. If you need to conduct the research independently, as in a thesis or dissertation, you may need to narrow your study down to the qualitative component. However, be wary of letting your methods drive your research questions! You have 2 alternatives. You may either collaborate with a quantitative researcher or learn quantitative methods and conduct your original study alone.

PRACTICAL CONSIDERATIONS

Now that you understand the arguments made against qualitative research and methods of mixing the qualitative and quantitative research paradigms, consider this practical advice. We have observed that when conducting studies, students often overlook small details that could make the process much more successful and enjoyable if included.

Preparing for Data Collection

In order to be efficient and effective, you must carefully prepare to collect data. We suggest that you pack your research bag ahead of time with the following items to be both effective and efficient:

- Interview and/or observation guide. Bring several unmarked copies for recording your notes.
- Omnidirectional microphone. This instrument picks up all voices, which is especially critical when conducting focus groups in which sounds come from different directions.
- Audio-recording device. Pack a portable USB charger or plenty of new batteries. Most phones or digital recorders now have a great deal of memory that lets you save more than one interview. Several phone apps are available to capture recordings on your device. Here are a couple that we or colleagues of ours have experience with:
  - TapeACall Pro (TelTech) is an app that allows you to record any phone calls. It is said to be simple to use and allows audio files to be uploaded to a cloud storage site such as Dropbox or Microsoft Azure.
  - NoNotes also allows you to save audio files to the cloud for storage or send them via email. This app allows you to record incoming or outgoing calls. NoNotes also contains an option for transcription services, making this quite a versatile app.
- Address or directions to the data collection site. This item is self-explanatory. Prepare an alternative route in case of construction or bad traffic.
- Video-recording device. This device is helpful for conducting observations. Make sure to obtain permission from participants before recording. Check that the tool has adequate storage capabilities. Pack extension cords, portable charger, and/or extra batteries.

- Contact information. Bring a phone number for your participant or primary contact at the site in case you are late or need to reschedule.
- Informed consent forms. Bring several unmarked copies for participants.
- Clipboard or something sturdy on which to write. Your writing must be legible, and the site may not provide a table or other hard surface.
- Appropriate attire. Consider your site and participants and dress to fit in, not stand out.
- Blank paper and writing utensil. You may desire an additional method for recording information.
- Photo identification. It is embarrassing and inconvenient to be turned away from your collection site because you lack the proper identification.

? *I am a graduate student with a very tight budget. Do I need to purchase all my research equipment personally?*

All research comes at a cost and you must create a budget. However, ask your institution, advisor, and colleagues if they have items you can borrow before you buy anything. Your institution may also have funding available for research expenses. Start asking for help early in the research process.

After packing your bag with the essentials for data collection, consider bringing duplicates of certain items in case something goes wrong. Think of these extra items like insurance: You may not use it when you have it, but when you don't have it, you need it!

- Bring extra portable chargers and/or batteries that will work with your equipment.
- Recording device. If possible, bring at least one extra device to record your interview or observation.
- Writing utensils. You can never have too many!
- Consent forms. You may come across another potential interviewee. Be ready to take advantage of this situation and have additional consent forms available.

Your bag is packed, and you are ready to go. Before leaving, please consider these tips that we learned from the school of hard knocks:

- Practice, practice, practice. Rehearse conducting interviews and setting up your equipment. Setting up always takes longer than you think, but the process will run more smoothly if you know what you're doing.
- Learn how to use your equipment. You must thoroughly understand the intricacies of your equipment. Do you have the widget that opens the battery compartment of the camera? Do you know where the camera's battery compartment is? Do you know where to plug in the microphone? Does your equipment have a separate power source?
- Assign pseudonyms carefully. If you intend to let participants select their own pseudonyms, you must have a plan for matching the pseudonyms with the participants' names in case you want to conduct additional interviews.
- Arrange a suitable interview location ahead of time. Don't assume that your participant will select the best venue for your needs. Visit the interview site ahead of time if possible, or arrive early enough to make necessary adjustments.

Conducting Data Collection

Although we have presented information for data collection earlier in this text, here are some additional practical tips to remember:

- Show appreciation for the participant's time.
- Be calm and professional at all times. This is not the time to project your opinions, try to be funny, or pretend to be something you are not.
- Make eye contact with your participant.
- Convey that the information you are collecting is important.
- Take your time. If you rush yourself, you will likely forget something. Take a deep breath and be systematic in your approach.

Following Up

- Thank your participants. Hand-write and send legible thank-you notes to everyone who assisted your process. You can also provide a typed acknowledgement of participation and time commitment for your participants' files or portfolios.
- Practice self-talk while leaving the site. Have a recorded conversation with yourself on the way back from the research site to capture your immediate thoughts about your experience. This recording of your initial reactions helps your reflection process.
- Secure your data. You will probably need your research bag for data collection again, so check the equipment and then repack it. However, you must remove your data from the bag immediately, back it up or make copies, and then store it in a secure place. You may never leave your data in a place where others could access it, whether intentionally or unintentionally. This is the contract you entered into with your institutional review board, and you must abide by it.
- Begin transcriptions promptly. The process of transcribing interviews or typing up observations always takes longer than you think it will, so start early. The longer you wait to begin, the more imposing the task will seem. Again, back your transcriptions up electronically and store them in a secure place. Do not use a hard drive, which could easily crash, as your sole storage unit.

Should you save the audio files you can choose to transcribe these yourself or have these professionally transcribed. Many companies are available for transcription services. As mentioned, NoNotes has this service as an option in the app. Other companies that we have used include TranscribeMe! (www.transcribeme.com) and Trint (https://trint.com), both of which allow for uploading of audio files for transcription purposes. Be sure to include the steps of recording and transcription services into your institutional review board approval process.

Using Software for Qualitative Research

Chapter 3 explains the general steps of qualitative analysis. Many researchers approach analysis manually by tracking coded concepts from transcripts along with quotes on a Microsoft Excel sheet and then organizing them into themes or categories. Some researchers use concept maps or word-processing files to organize their data and display emergent themes. Others use programs known as *computer-assisted qualitative data analysis software* (CAQDAS) to organize and sort textual data. In a study by Rodik and Primorac,[2] they discovered that many researchers adopt CAQDAS because it is perceived to make the analysis more systematic, convenient, and easier. Additionally, there is a perception that it lends credibility to the analysis.

Next we provide information on common software. However, we must emphasize that although software helps you organize your coded concepts, and store and retrieve your data, it will not interpret it for you.[3] The researcher is the instrument for data collection and analysis. Webb[4] suggests that novice qualitative researchers use a manual technique rather than a CAQDAS program. Once you have gained experience with the interpretive process, you may progress to software programs.

Many programs exist, but we share the following 3 here because either we or our colleagues have successfully used them. We don't believe that any one program is better than another. Because each program has particular nuances and ways of organizing data, you must choose the one you feel most comfortable with. Although choice of software is largely a matter of personal preference, graduate students and new faculty members usually use the programs made available by their departments.

- MAXQDA (VERBI) provides a platform for researchers to analyze non-numerical data and allows for sorting, structuring, and analyzing material, including image and audio files. Essentially, the software allows you to import the data and then transcribe these into the program. The platform also allows for memos and visualizing relationships between categories of data. For more information, visit www.maxqda.com/what-is-computer-assisted-data-analysis

- NVivo (QSR International) software allows researchers to import, code, and organize transcripts and documents that contain tables and figures. The program's features let researchers keep memos and display relationships between coded concepts. Go to www.qsrinternational.com/nvivo/nvivo-products for more information.

- Whereas the first 2 programs are desktop based, the Coding Analysis Toolkit (Texifter) is a web-based platform that is open source, meaning it is free to use. The platform allows for coding of transcripts as well as creating analytical memos. Further, Coding Analysis Toolkit allows for multiple analysts (coders) and has a function that allows you to determine the level of agreement, or inter-rater reliability. You can find more information on this platform at https://cat.texifter.com

I do not have time to simultaneously conduct my study and learn to use computerized software. What should I do?

You should never attempt these 2 tasks at the same time. You should master a computerized software package before you even turn on a microphone or begin collecting data. If this is not the case, then manually analyzing your data will actually be more efficient.

PRESENTING YOUR RESEARCH PLAN

Having read this far, you are likely thinking of presenting your research study either to a committee as part of a thesis or dissertation or to an agency to receive funding for your study. Here we present some practical information related to advanced planning for your research.

In addition to the main body of the proposal, you should include various appendices for all reviewers, containing such items as interview guides, informed consent forms, and observation instruments. Placing each of these in a separate appendix lets you share the information without substantially interrupting the flow of your writing. If you are writing a grant proposal, your appendices may also include letters of support from critical parties (eg, department chair, advisor, dean) and evidence of supplemental funding. Table 11-1 presents an overview of contents that are necessary in a proposal and displays the similarities and differences between an academic proposal and a grant proposal.

We suggest including an appendix with a timeline for completion of your study, which is beneficial even when it is not required. The timeline serves several key purposes. First, it shows that you have thought through each step of the research process and determined a realistic time frame for completion. Second, it allows the members of your committee to check their availability. For example, if committee members are scheduled for a sabbatical at a time when you are most likely to need their expertise, you must begin rescheduling or looking for replacements. Third, if your proposal is for funding, the timeline will help the funding agency ensure that your study will meet the dissemination deadlines often associated with grants.

When creating your timeline, remember to invite Mr. Murphy, lest he appear as an unwelcome guest! Locke, Spirduso, and Silverman[5] capture this concept when they state, "Murphy's Law dictates that, in the conduct of research, if anything can go wrong, it probably will." In other words, with careful consideration in the proposal stage, you should be able to anticipate most of the problems that could arise in the course of your study. We suggest using a teaching strategy called *if-then*.[6] Examine each step of your research process and try to plan for all eventualities. For example, *if* the person transcribing my interviews changes the anticipated deadline for completion, *then* I will (1) transcribe them myself or (2) hire an undergraduate student to assist. Consider how each potential problem would affect your timeline.

You must include a budget for a grant proposal. Some funding agencies require the inclusion of the budget in the main body of the document, whereas others prefer it in an appendix. Wherever you place it, be sure to give the budget the full attention it deserves. Don't estimate the cost of items, but rather check out options and provide quotes. Obtain the latest information regarding standard budgetary items, such as mileage rates, transcription costs, and registration fees. Be sure that the items listed in the budget are eligible for funding. If they are not, seek supplemental funding for those items and provide evidence of that funding. In our experience, funding agencies, particularly for internal or local grants, are often more receptive to proposals that have already established some financial backing.

	Table 11-1	
CRITICAL COMPONENTS: SIMILARITIES AND DIFFERENCES BETWEEN ACADEMIC AND GRANT PROPOSALS		
COMPONENT	**ACADEMIC (THESIS OR DISSERTATION)**	**GRANT**
Introduction	• Conceptual framework • Statement of the problem • Purpose statement • Research questions • Significance of the study • Author's perspective • Definition of terms	• Conceptual framework • Statement of the problem • Purpose statement • Research questions • Significance of the study • Links to mission of funding agency
Literature review	Should be extensive, covering critical articles and presenting interpretations to support current study	Often a short, condensed version of an extensive review that includes critical articles to support current research
Methods	• Participants • Sampling • Procedures • Data collection • Data analysis • Ensuring trustworthiness	• Participants • Sampling • Procedures • Data collection • Data analysis • Ensuring trustworthiness • Anticipated outcomes (where will results be disseminated?)
Timeline	Needed for plans to complete the study (helps establish feasibility with committee members)	Needed to assure funding agency that you will adhere to deadlines and complete the project in a timely manner *(continued)*

TABLE 11-1 (CONTINUED)		
CRITICAL COMPONENTS: SIMILARITIES AND DIFFERENCES BETWEEN ACADEMIC AND GRANT PROPOSALS		
COMPONENT	**ACADEMIC (THESIS OR DISSERTATION)**	**GRANT**
Budget		Must be clear and items must match the funding available from the agency (always check carefully to determine whether items such as travel, conference registrations, and equipment can be funded)
Support/ matching funds		If possible, show evidence of matching funds or supplemental funding
References	Must be included to give adequate credit to literature that has guided your conceptualization of the study	Must be included to give adequate credit to literature that has guided your conceptualization of the study
Appendices	• Informed consent • Observation/interview guides	• Informed consent • Observation/interview guides • Letters from advisor/dean/chair • Obtain letters of support from critical parties (eg, advisor, chair, dean)

With respect to presenting your research ideas, we would be remiss if we did not address critical issues related to orally presenting your proposed study. Indeed, you will commonly present your study to a committee before conducting a thesis or dissertation. Consider the following dos and don'ts when preparing for an oral presentation.

Do

- Prepare a script with content related to all 3 sections (introduction, literature review, and methods).
- Practice, revise. Practice, revise. Practice, revise!
- Maintain eye contact with your audience (one suggestion to help with this is to have your script in large font on the top third of every page).
- Construct a slide presentation that highlights key points.
- Provide handouts for committee members.
- Anticipate questions and draft answers ahead of time.
- Be concise when describing the literature.
- Be prepared to make changes. The job of your committee members is to offer suggestions for improving your study.
- Be honest. It is all right to admit that you don't know the answer to a question.
- Be enthusiastic about your study.
- Dress and act professionally.

Don't

- Act defensive.
- Simply read your slide presentation aloud without any explanation.
- Explain every single study you have read like a verbal string of pearls.
- Get carried away, speaking beyond the given time frame.
- Forget to thank the members of your committee and audience.

Do I need to write a proposal if I am not required to present one?

Yes! You must complete a detailed proposal even if you are not required to present it. Remember, if you fail to plan, you should plan to fail.

Locating Resources

The following online resources will help you answer questions as you move forward in your journey with qualitative research:

- The Qualitative Report has many resources, including an academic journal, news updates, and resource links. For information related to practicing, teaching, and assessing the quality of qualitative research, go to https://tqr.nova.edu
- QualPage contains many resources related to qualitative research, including a variety of research approaches, reports, digital tools, journals and publishers, and other resources. Go to https://qualpage.com to access the site.

- Cochrane Methods—Qualitative and Implementation Methods Group. The Cochrane Qualitative Research Methods Group (CQRMG) has a website to develop awareness of qualitative research for health care professions. Their focus is on methodological guidance and the synthesis of qualitative evidence to inform practice. The CQRMG site explains the role of qualitative evidence in health care and provides information for reviewing qualitative research. Visit https://methods.cochrane.org/qi/welcome for more information.

SUMMARY

This chapter provided closing advice, including how to counter arguments against qualitative research, practical advice for collecting data, and where to locate some helpful resources. Embrace the role of educator, advocate for qualitative research, and consider the practical necessities of your task as a researcher. Access and read about recent developments in the research community. Finally, prepare to enjoy your future as a qualitative researcher!

CONTINUE YOUR EDUCATIONAL JOURNEY

LEARN THROUGH ACTIVITY

1. Conduct an Internet search for useful information that has been updated in the past year using the following key terms: qualitative research, qualitative data analysis, and interpretive research.
2. Search the Internet for information about 2 software packages for qualitative research other than those previously cited. Compare and contrast the programs.

CHECK YOUR KNOWLEDGE

1. Which of the following is a common misconception about qualitative research?
   a. It is not rigorous.
   b. It is scientifically based.
   c. It gains insight and understanding.
   d. It is objective.
   e. b and c
2. It is recommended that a novice researcher not use computer assisted qualitative analysis software.
   a. True
   b. False

3. Although qualitative research findings cannot be generalized, they can be transferable to similar contexts.
   a. True
   b. False

4. The positive aspect of a qualitative research software package is that it will literally analyze the data for you.
   a. True
   b. False

5. After collecting data, your first step must be to secure and back up your files.
   a. True
   b. False

THINK ABOUT IT

1. You are debating the value of qualitative research with a colleague. After some time, you realize that no matter how you articulate your stance, your colleague will always consider your research inferior. How do you manage this situation?

2. You have conducted a mixed methods study and submitted your manuscript for review. Your reviewer considers mixed methods studies weaker than pure, single-method studies. How should you respond?

3. After arriving at your interview site, you realize you forgot your informed consent forms. What options do you have now?

MAKE A STRETCH

These readings will expand your knowledge on using qualitative research software:

- Evers JC. Current issues in qualitative data analysis software (QDAS): a user and developer perspective. *Qual Rep.* 2018;23(13):61-73.
- Locke LF, Spirduso WW, Silverman SJ. *Proposals That Work: A Guide for Planning Dissertation and Grant Proposals.* 6th ed. Thousand Oaks, CA: Sage; 2013.
- Schwandt TA. *The SAGE Dictionary of Qualitative Inquiry.* 4th ed. Thousand Oaks, CA: Sage; 2015.
- Wolski U. The history of the development and propagation of QDA software. *Qual Rep.* 2018;23(13):6-20.

REFERENCES

1. Dingwall R. Don't mind him—he's from Barcelona: qualitative methods in health studies. In Daly J, MacDonald I, Willis E, eds. *Researching Health Care: Design, Dilemmas, Disciplines.* London, England: Tavistoch/Routledge; 1992:161-175.

2. Rodik P, Primorac J. To use or not to use: computer-assisted qualitative data analysis software usage among early-career sociologists in Croatia. *Qual Soc Res.* http://www.qualitative-research.net/index.php/fqs/article/view/2221. Published 2015. Accessed June 25, 2019.

3. Morison M, Moir J. The role of computer software in the analysis of qualitative data: efficient clerk, research assistant, or Trojan horse? *J Adv Nurs.* 1998;28(1):106-116.

4. Webb C. Analysing qualitative data: computerized and other approaches. *J Advanced Nurs.* 1999;29(2):323-330.

5. Locke LF, Spirduso WW, Silverman SJ. *Proposals That Work: A Guide for Planning Dissertation and Grant Proposals.* 4th ed. Thousand Oaks, CA: Sage; 2000.

6. Tjeerdsma BL. If-then statements help novice teachers deal with the unexpected. *JOPERD.* 1995;66(9):22-24.

Answers to
Check Your Knowledge

PART ONE

Chapter 1

1. b
2. c
3. b
4. a
5. d
6. d

Chapter 2

1. e
2. b
3. a
4. c
5. b
6. b
7. e

PART TWO

Chapter 3

1. b
2. e
3. a
4. a
5. c
6. b

Chapter 4

1. a
2. b
3. c
4. a
5. c

Chapter 5

1. b
2. a
3. d
4. e
5. d

Chapter 6

1. b
2. c
3. d
4. b
5. f

Pitney WA, Parker J, Mazerolle Singe S, Potteiger K.
Qualitative Research in the Health Professions (pp 165-166).
© 2020 Taylor & Francis Group.

PART THREE

Chapter 7

1. a
2. c
3. a
4. b
5. b
6. a
7. d
8. c

Chapter 8

1. a
2. c
3. a
4. d
5. a
6. d

Chapter 9

1. a
2. d
3. b
4. b
5. a
6. d

Chapter 10

1. b
2. a
3. c
4. c
5. a

Chapter 11

1. a
2. a
3. a
4. b
5. a

Financial Disclosures

Dr. Christianne M. Eason has no financial or proprietary interest in the materials presented herein.

Dr. Jenny Parker has no financial or proprietary interest in the materials presented herein.

Dr. William A. Pitney has no financial or proprietary interest in the materials presented herein.

Dr. Stephanie Mazerolle Singe has no financial or proprietary interest in the materials presented herein.

Dr. Kelly Potteiger has no financial or proprietary interest in the materials presented herein.

Index

Printed in the United States
by Baker & Taylor Publisher Services